DATE DUE

Locomotor Training

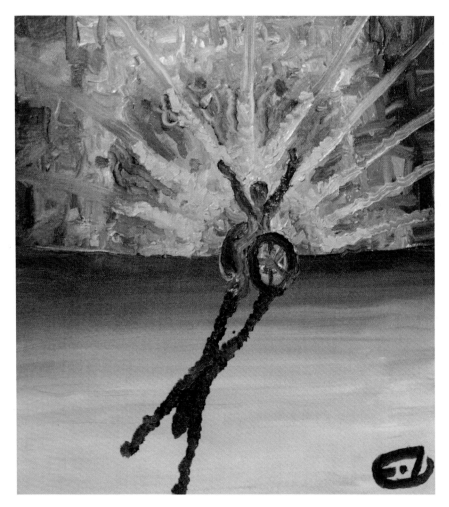

"Shadow" © Tobias Forrest

Locomotor Training

Principles and Practice

Susan J. Harkema, PhD
Kentucky Spinal Cord Injury Research Center
Department of Neurological Surgery
University of Louisville and
Frazier Rehab Institute
Louisville, KY

Andrea L. Behrman, PhD, PT, FAPTA
Physical Therapy Department
University of Florida, and
Research Health Scientist
Brain Rehabilitation Research Center
Malcom Randall VA Medical Center
Gainesville, FL

Hugues Barbeau, PhD
School of Physical and Occupational Therapy
McGill University
Montréal, Québec
Canada

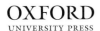

OXFORD
UNIVERSITY PRESS

OXFORD
UNIVERSITY PRESS

Oxford University Press, Inc., publishes works that further
Oxford University's objective of excellence
in research, scholarship, and education.

Oxford   New York
Auckland   Cape Town   Dar es Salaam   Hong Kong   Karachi
Kuala Lumpur   Madrid   Melbourne   Mexico City   Nairobi
New Delhi   Shanghai   Taipei   Toronto

With offices in
Argentina   Austria   Brazil   Chile   Czech Republic   France   Greece
Guatemala   Hungary   Italy   Japan   Poland   Portugal   Singapore
South Korea   Switzerland   Thailand   Turkey   Ukraine   Vietnam

Published by Oxford University Press, Inc.
198 Madison Avenue, New York, New York 10016
www.oup.com

Oxford is a registered trademark of Oxford University Press

Library of Congress Cataloging-in-Publication Data

Harkema, Susan.
Locomotor training : principles and practice / Susan Harkema,
Andrea L. Behrman, Hugues Barbeau.
    p.; cm.

Includes bibliographical references and index.
ISBN 978-0-19-534208-6
1. Movement therapy. 2. Spinal cord—Wounds and injuries—Patients—Rehabilitation.
3. Cerebrovascular disease—Patients—Rehabilitation. 4. Human locomotion.
I. Behrman, Andrea L. II. Barbeau, Hugues, 1953- III. Title.
[DNLM: 1. Walking–physiology. 2. Locomotion–physiology.
3. Spinal Cord Injuries–rehabilitation. 4. Stroke–rehabilitation. WE 103 H282L 2011]

RC489.M66H37 2011
615.8'2–dc22   2010014918

9 8 7 6 5 4 3 2 1
Printed in the United States of America
on acid-free paper

In memory of Gayle Sims Behrman Jaster and Merrell Sue Harkema.

In appreciation to the many individuals with neurologic dysfunction who have taught us and continue to teach us by their courage and experiences.

In appreciation to the therapists and activity-based technicians of the Christopher and Dana Reeve NeuroRecovery Network and researchers who have contributed their knowledge and expertise.

Foreword

Anyone who is thinking about postural and locomotor training to regain function following a spinal cord injury and probably other injuries related to deficits involving these motor tasks, would be wise to study the text *Locomotor Training: Principles and Practice* by Harkema, Behrman, and Barbeau. The principal reasons for this are threefold. First, the three authors have been at the forefront from the beginning of the new realization that the human spinal cord exhibits some of the plasticity in neuro-muscular function that has been demonstrated so clearly in animal models of spinal cord injury. They have been at the forefront at the clinical and at the basic level and the techniques that seem to be the most effective in locomotor training have evolved from ideas and concepts that have emerged from each of these authors. This book has taken advantage of the combined expertise of the three. The second reason for paying close attention to the contents of this text is that it provides a brief background which describes the conceptual basis of the techniques developed from animal experimentation that are being applied in the clinic. Thirdly, these three authors have learned that an understanding of these basic concepts and the recognition that what appear to be subtle techniques in training an individual with an injury are really not so subtle. Paying attention to these details in training techniques, based on years of experience, is likely to improve the chances of more favorable functional outcomes. Finally, it would be important to recognize the limitations and the issues as described in the text so that one understands where there are convincing data which provide a basis for a given procedure, versus when there remains a question as to its efficacy.

V. Reggie Edgerton, PhD
Los Angeles, CA

Acknowledgments

Thank you to the Fondation pour la recherche sur la moelle épinière; National Institute of Neurological Disorders and Stroke, National Center for Medical Rehabilitation Research (National Institute of Child Health and Human Development) of the National Institutes of Health; Christopher and Dana Reeve Foundation; Craig H. Neilsen Foundation; and the Department of Veterans Affairs Rehabilitation, Research and Development, and the Veterans Affairs Brain Rehabilitation Research Center for their continuous support. We thank Jessica Hillyer for her careful review and editing of the chapters.

The following sources for photographs are also acknowledged:

Chapter 3

Figure 3-1: Photographs provided by the University of Florida, Department of Physical Therapy, Gainesville, FL.
Figure 3-2: Photographs provided by Christopher and Dana Reeve Foundation (CDRF) NeuroRecovery Network Boston, MA, and Frazier Rehab Institute, Louisville, KY.
Figure 3-3: Photograph provided by CDRF NeuroRecovery Network at The Institute for Rehabilitation and Research, Houston, TX.

Chapter 4

All photographs provided by Department of Physical Therapy, University of Florida, and VA Brain Rehabilitation Research Center, Malcom Randall VA Medical Center, Gainesville, FL.

Chapter 5

All photographs provided by CDRF NeuroRecovery Network at The Ohio State University Medical Center, Columbus, OH."

Chapter 6

Figures 6-1, 6-2, 6-6, 6-7, and 6-8: Photographs provided by CDRF NeuroRecovery Network at Shepherd Center, Atlanta, GA.
Figures 6-3 and 6-5: Photographs provided by CDRF NeuroRecovery Network, Magee Rehabilitation Hospital, Philadelphia, PA.

Figures 6-4, 6-9, and 6-11: Photographs provided by Department of Physical Therapy, University of Florida and VA Brain Rehabilitation Research Center, Malcom Randall VA Medical Center, Gainesville, FL.
Figures 6-10 and 6-12: Photographs provided by CDRF NeuroRecovery Network, The Institute for Rehabilitation and Research, Houston, TX.

Chapter 7

Figures 7-1–7-12, 7-14, 7-16, 7-17, 7-20–7-23, 7-25, 7-27, 7-28, and 7-30: Photographs provided by CDRF NeuroRecovery Network, Magee Rehabilitation Hospital, Philadelphia, PA.
Figures 7-13, 7-15, 7-18, and 7-19: Photographs provided by CDRF NeuroRecovery Network, Kessler Institute for Rehabilitation, West Orange, NJ.
Figures 7-24, 7-26, and 7-29: Photographs provided by CDRF NeuroRecovery Network, The Institute for Rehabilitation and Research, Houston, TX.

Chapter 8

All photographs provided by CDRF NeuroRecovery Network, Magee Rehabilitation Hospital, Philadelphia, PA.

Contents

Locomotor Training

1

Evidence-Based Practice and Activity-Based Therapy for Recovery of Posture, Standing, and Walking

Chapter Outline

Chapter Objectives

The objectives of Chapter 1 are to:

1. Understand the history of rehabilitative approaches after neurologic injury or disease.
2. Understand the history of rehabilitative approaches for spinal cord injury and stroke.
3. Describe the gait deficiencies following spinal cord injury and stroke.
4. Discuss evidence-based practice.

Summary

This chapter reviews physical rehabilitation for posture, standing, and walking from an historical perspective and provides a context for the emergence of Locomotor Training as an activity-based therapy after spinal cord injury (SCI) and stroke by implementing evidence-based practice. This chapter is not intended to be a comprehensive review of the functional consequences after injury or insult or a review of all the available rehabilitation strategies for SCI or stroke. Rather, it is intended to be a discussion within the framework of introducing Locomotor Training as a new strategy to augment already successful therapeutic approaches. The review presented here is not a discourse of accepted clinical practices but is a summary of evidence from studies in individuals after SCI or stroke related to functional deficits affecting mobility, posture, standing, and walking.

Rehabilitation of Walking After Neurologic Injury or Disease: A Historical Perspective

SCI and stroke modify the sensorimotor, musculoskeletal, autonomic, and central nervous systems, generally limiting physical activity and leading to secondary complications that affect health and quality of life (Go et al., 1995; Noreau & Shephard, 1995). Historically, rehabilitation after stroke has predominantly targeted reducing spasticity, reducing abnormal movement patterns, and providing sensorimotor facilitation to activate weak muscles. In comparison, rehabilitation after SCI has concentrated on strengthening the muscles above the level of the lesion to compensate for weak or paralyzed muscles below the injury site but has limited focus on strategies that would restore function below the level of the lesion.

These compensatory strategies were developed in part based on the clinical reaction to polio, a health epidemic that affected millions of people and resulted in paralysis and weakness leading to debilitating effects on the individual's ability to walk, breathe, or use his or her arms (Quiben, 2006). This overwhelming epidemic led rehabilitation specialists to develop compensation strategies to allow individuals to function adequately in their daily lives more than restorative strategies when there was little hope for neurologic recovery (Sharrard, 1955). Functional goals such as standing and walking were achieved with the use of braces and assistive devices (Quiben, 2006). In cases of severe paralysis, long leg braces were used to support paralyzed legs, which permitted the achievement of standing. Assistive devices, such as forearm crutches, were used to provide the balance and momentum needed for walking so that individuals using "brace walking" literally vaulted over crutches to advance their limbs.

These strategies led to the functional recovery of upright mobility in many of those with polio; however, this type of mobility required entirely new movement strategies based on using unaffected muscles to compensate for those affected by the disease. The alternative strategy was to forego upright mobility completely and use a wheelchair. While assistive devices afforded ambulation, the functional task of walking as known and experienced prior to the onset of polio was neither restored nor recovered by the therapeutic intervention. Therefore, individuals were able to function in their home and community by taking advantage of compensatory strategies even though weakness and paralysis persisted. These approaches were then translated to other neurologic disorders, including SCI and stroke.

Various approaches to physical neurorehabilitation have developed since the polio era, in which therapists apply the theoretical models of motor control and clinical experience to maximize outcomes following neurologic injury or disease. These strategies include proprioceptive neuromuscular facilitation (Adler et al., 1999), neurodevelopmental treatment (Davies, 1985), impairment-based therapies (Krebs et al., 2008), spasticity-reducing strategies (Boviatsis et al., 2005), part-to-whole training (Schmidt & Lee, 1999), and the use of braces/assistive devices to compensate for neuromuscular deficits and afford mobility (Somers, 2001). Principles of motor learning and theories of motor control had a dominant influence on physical rehabilitation in the 1990s (Schmidt & Lee, 1999; Shumway-Cook & Woolacot, 1995), providing strategies to enhance learning via manipulation of feedback, knowledge of results, and conditions of practice. Therapists were introduced to concepts to enhance skill acquisition for patients relearning daily tasks, while also learning new compensatory movement patterns to accomplish everyday functions. The field of motor learning provided a new perspective on the therapy session and on how it could be designed to more effectively promote improved performance, retention of new skills, and transfer or generalization of skills. Massed practice, variable practice, and part-to-whole practice became models for task practice during therapy sessions.

The field of motor control provided theoretical frameworks for the retraining or acquisition of motor skills after neurologic injury to meet the demands of specific tasks. One such framework incorporates a systems theory of motor control and uses a task-oriented approach (Shumway-Cook & Woollacott, 1995) for application to clinical practice. Motor control is viewed as an emergence of an interaction between the individual, the task, and the environment in which the task is being executed. Broadly, the tasks carried out by individuals include postural control, mobility functions, and upper extremity control; however, compensation strategies remain an integral aspect of the rehabilitation process.

Recovery of Posture and Walking After Spinal Cord Injury

Approximately 1,275,000 individuals in the United States and 41,000 individuals in Canada are living with the consequences of SCI. The incidence of SCI is estimated to be over 12,000 new cases annually in the United States and 1,400 new cases in Canada (Gibson et al., 2009). The average age at injury today is 48 years; it was 40 years in 2005 and 29 years between 1973 and 1979. Enhanced emphasis on emergency medical care at the site of the accident and other interventions has resulted in a change in the extent of SCI: previously most injuries were complete, but now the majority are incomplete injuries. Statistics have shown that 52.6% of injuries are incomplete (tetraplegia, 34%; paraplegia, 19%), while only 47% are complete injuries (tetraplegia, 18%; paraplegia, 23%). Methylprednisolone was introduced in the 1990s as a drug to minimize the secondary effects of injury, and although its efficacy is still being debated, it is considered to have contributed to a shift towards improved recovery after SCI. This shift has increased the potential for walking recovery with sparing of sensorimotor function below the level of the lesion (Stover et al., 1999); however, physical rehabilitation has remained focused on compensation.

Functional Deficits After Spinal Cord Injury

There are many functional deficits in the locomotion of individuals following SCI. For clinically complete and severely injured incomplete individuals, locomotion has been unattainable. Individuals with motor complete SCI exhibit paralysis of the musculature below the level of the lesion. They are unable to voluntarily activate trunk and leg muscles below the spinal cord lesion. Deficits or complete loss of sensation and proprioception disrupt sensory feedback concerning posture and limb position, pressure, or tactile information. Restoration of pre-injury ambulation ability and standing is not expected and is not a goal of rehabilitation. Passive standing and mobility are achieved by alternative strategies and devices.

Though individuals with motor incomplete SCI have greater potential to achieve walking, few individuals achieve a full return to normal ambulatory function. Those who do achieve ambulation walk with a slow, asymmetrical gait pattern, have balance difficulties, depend on assistive devices for support, and use braces to compensate for weakness or paralysis. The first striking difference observed in the gait of ambulatory individuals with incomplete SCI is reduced walking speed. In a retrospective review, speed data were pooled from 162 individuals with incomplete SCI across 20 studies (Barbeau et al., 1998), showing a wide spectrum of walking speed abilities, ranging from total incapacity to near-normal speed. Next, the kinematic pattern at the trunk, hip, knee, and ankle joints reveals a different profile between individuals with SCI and those without injury when both groups are compared at their natural walking speeds (Pepin et al., 2003a, 2003b). Those with incomplete SCI walk with more ankle dorsiflexion during the initial double-stance period, with less plantarflexion during the push-off component. Flexion of the knee at initial contact is accentuated, although it is reduced during swing (Barbeau et al., 1999). Besides being of lesser amplitude, the peak ankle plantarflexion during push-off and the peak knee flexion during swing are reached later. Finally, in the SCI population, the maximal hip extension tends to be less.

Joint stiffness, including the relative contribution of the stretch reflex and the intrinsic properties of the ankle extensors in normal and spastic subjects, has been studied by several groups (Dietz et al., 1981; Dietz & Berger, 1983; Sinkjaer & Magnussen, 1994; Thilmann et al., 1991). An increase in the reflex gain and a decrease in inhibition during the swing phase have been reported in individuals with incomplete SCI (Fung & Barbeau, 1994; Sinkjaer et al., 1996; Yang et al., 1991). These findings suggest that increases in both the reflex gain and the non-reflex torque could contribute to the increased stiffness of the ankle joint seen in individuals with incomplete SCI during walking. Hence, both alterations in central mechanisms and changes in intrinsic properties of the muscle fibers could be responsible for the increased stiffness and for the decreased walking speed (Mirbagheri et al., 2001).

In addition, a comparison of the kinetics (moment and mechanical power) of individuals with incomplete SCI and of non-injured individuals walking at natural speeds presents significant differences at the ankle, knee, and hip joints. The individuals with SCI have smaller plantarflexor moments generated at the ankle joint during terminal stance, and the use of short leg braces accentuates this weakness. At the knee joint, individuals with incomplete SCI have a higher flexion moment at initial contact and during terminal stance. On the other hand, they present a lower extension moment during mid-stance. Also, individuals with incomplete SCI exhibit an increase in the flexor moment at the hip during mid-stance and a decrease in hip extensor moment during terminal stance. This results in an important difference (decrease) in energy generation. At the knee joint, lower energy absorption during loading response is also observed (Nadeau et al., 1999).

The electromyogram (EMG) of lower limb muscles during walking reveals alterations in both timing and amplitude in individuals with SCI compared to uninjured individuals (Fung & Barbeau, 1994). Co-activation of muscle activity at proximal and distal joints is often reported in individuals with incomplete SCI (Fung & Barbeau, 1994). Further abnormal activation of the soleus muscle, including a broadened and flattened EMG profile with an early activation and clonus during the stance phase, is commonly seen in early stance.

In summary, individuals with incomplete SCI exhibit dysfunction in most of the critical events of the gait cycle. Weakness of the knee extensors modifies the gait cycle during the loading phase and weakness of the ankle plantarflexors corresponds to changes in terminal stance and pre-swing phases (Bajd et al., 1997). The initial and mid-swing phases are affected by changes in the passive and reflex stiffness of the ankle plantarflexors as well as weakness of the ankle dorsiflexors (Dietz et al., 1981). Finally, terminal swing is affected by a decrease in angular velocity generated by the weakness of the hip flexors. This resultant behavior is a product of intersegmental dynamics that are dependent on the velocity of the movement (Hoy & Zernicke, 1986; Wisleder et al., 1990).

In humans, uphill walking is a demanding task that requires specific modifications in the trunk and the pelvis and in lower limb movements (Lange et al., 1996; Wall et al., 1981) and muscle activation patterns (Brandell, 1977; Lange et al., 1996; Simonsen et al., 1995). As the walking grade increases, more propulsion has to be generated from the lower limbs (Brandell, 1977) and postural adjustments must be performed to maintain equilibrium. Following SCI, the basic locomotor pattern is altered (Barbeau et al., 1998), and the ability to adapt to changes in the environment could be affected. For example, increasing the treadmill slope from 0 to 15 degrees induces a gradual increase in hip and knee flexion and in ankle dorsiflexion from late swing through the stance phase, and the vertical displacement of the greater trochanter is stable across grades in all uninjured subjects. In individuals with incomplete SCI, however, lower limb motions do not show consistent patterns of adaptation. Individuals who are unable to achieve the steepest slope (15%) show only increased hip flexion in early stance combined with elevation of the greater trochanter (hip hiking) during the swing phase in all walking conditions. This hip hiking is used, in part, to compensate for the decrease or the absence of the tibialis anterior activity during the swing phase (Leroux et al., 1999).

Researchers also investigated the contribution of the trunk and pelvis during inclined walking in uninjured subjects and those with incomplete SCI (Leroux et al., 2002, 2006). Briefly, their results show the importance of trunk and pelvic segments in the postural adaptation to inclined walking. Trunk and pelvic movements do not seem to participate directly in the generation or absorption of energy required for walking up and down slopes. Total angular excursions are consistent across walking grades in sagittal and transverse planes and vary to a small degree in the frontal plane. However, modifications in trunk and pelvic vertical alignment allowed lower limbs to perform the most efficient patterns of movements during uphill and downhill walking. Thus, the researchers propose that trunk and pelvic postural modifications likely assist lower limbs when adapting to inclined walking (Ladouceur et al., 2003; Leroux et al., 2002, 2006). In SCI individuals the inability to control the trunk and pelvis contributes to the difficulty in successfully negotiating an incline.

Stepping over an obstacle is another locomotor task with greater demands and challenges to postural control when compared to steady-state walking on level ground. The anticipatory locomotor adjustments exhibited when stepping over obstacles shows a spectrum of adaptation capacities similar to walking speed and slope. The greater trochanter during quiet standing was used as a reference to measure the relative vertical displacements. Uninjured subjects increased both hip and knee flexion during early swing when encountering 5- and 30-mm obstacles. At the opposite end of the spectrum of adaptations, individuals with incomplete SCI are typically incapable of clearing small obstacles of only 5 mm. They do not adapt the trajectory of the fifth metatarsal during the obstructed condition (30 mm), showing that the unobstructed foot trajectory is insufficient to clear such a low-height obstacle. However, there are changes in the locomotor pattern with an elevation of the greater trochanter and a decrease in knee flexion at the initiation of the swing phase (Ladouceur et al., 2003). Therefore, different compensation strategies can be adopted by individuals with incomplete SCI, such as elevating the greater trochanter to adapt to increased speed, or increasing hip circumduction and/or knee flexion to clear obstacles.

Examples of other functional changes in the musculoskeletal system following neurologic insult are increased stiffness of the passive components of the ankle joint (Mirbagheri et al., 2001, 2002), increased fatigability and modification of the biochemical properties of motor units (Cope et al., 1986; Stein et al., 1991; Veltink et al., 2000; Yang et al., 1990), and a higher incidence of osteoporosis (Demirel et al., 1998; Garland et al., 1992; Wilmet et al., 1995). Furthermore, depending upon the level of the injury, there is a modification of the autonomic regulation system, including adaptations of the circulatory system and bladder, digestive, and sexual function (Hooker et al., 1993; Raymond et al., 1997; Yamamoto et al., 1999). SCI is also associated with changes within the central nervous system, such as weakness, hyperactive spinal reflexes (Dietz et al., 1981; Sinkjaer et al., 1996), muscle co-activation, and loss of sensory function (Fung & Barbeua, 1994; Sinkjaer et al., 1996; Yang et al., 1991). For individuals with clinically complete injury these complications tend to be more severe and debilitating, and after incomplete injuries these modifications contribute to deficits in walking and to postural problems related to bearing weight, maintaining balance, and developing propulsion.

Physical Rehabilitation After Spinal Cord Injury

The key factors that are considered before initiation of standard gait rehabilitation for individuals with SCI are voluntary motor control, range of motion, muscle tone, sensation, functional abilities, posture, skin integrity, and autonomic function (Behrman et al., 2009). The assessed voluntary function of the 10 key lower limb muscles (e.g., left and right hip flexors, knee extensors, ankle dorsiflexors, long toe extensors, and ankle plantarflexors) is used as a key predictor for potential of recovery of locomotion. In addition, upper limb strength is assessed for the availability of controlling balance assist and support devices. This assessment and the subsequent interpretation by the rehabilitation specialist usually determines the approach to reaching ambulatory functional goals and the level of effort that will be given toward neuromuscular recovery versus compensation approaches.

Historically, the predominant approach for rehabilitation for persons with SCI has been to compensate for the neuromuscular deficits caused by the injury (Halstead & Grimby, 1995; Sadowsky & McDonald, 2009; Whiteneck et al., 2009). Upper limbs can be used to compensate for the lack of trunk control and leg paralysis, allowing individuals with SCI to move their own body and to perform activities of daily living. Therapy targets strengthening the muscles above the level of the lesion. Leg braces are used to provide support when muscles are weak or paralyzed. For persons with complete or severe incomplete SCI, bracing is used to fully support the leg and sometimes assist at the hip joint and pelvis (e.g., long leg braces, LSU reciprocating gait orthoses). Strategies to ambulate include vaulting over supported limbs while weight-bearing through the arms with crutches using a swing-through gait pattern.

Assistive devices have been traditionally used to accomplish mobility (Sisto et al., 2008). A consequence of the many altered features of gait in individuals with incomplete SCI is an increase in the energy requirement necessary for ambulation, an issue for consideration when deciding on an assistive device. Melis and colleagues (1999) showed that individuals using walkers tend to walk slower than crutch users, who tend to walk slower than cane users. The opposite relationship exists for the maximal amount of force exerted on a walking aid during gait: walker users tend to place the most amount of force on their aid, cane users the least. These results suggest that walking speed might be related to maximal axial force, or that the limiting factor in the speed of an individual's gait might be, in fact, the type of walking aid itself. More recently, functional electrical stimulation (FES) has developed as an alternative orthosis, compensating for lack of voluntary activation of leg muscles for standing and walking (Bogataj et al., 1995; Ditunno & Scivoletto, 2009; Kirshblum, 2004; Stein et al., 1993). The FES orthosis can be used to provide dorsiflexion during the swing phase of the gait cycle or can provide gross flexion and extension when used as bilateral leg orthoses in lieu of long leg braces (e.g., ParaStep System). When these devices are removed, there is no therapeutic effect on the user's ability to move his or her legs or walk more easily. Thus, these devices achieve a mobility goal but do not restore neuromuscular function.

The wheelchair, manual or power, remains an optional and alternative means of daily mobility. Where wheelchair propulsion approximates the energy requirement of normal walking (Blessey, 1978), the energy cost of walking by individuals with incomplete SCI is higher than that for speed-matched walking by able-bodied participants (Stein et al., 1993), making upright mobility aids much more demanding. Movement strategies that take advantage of principles of physics (such as levers and momentum) and substitution via alternative muscle use (Behrman et al., 2006; Sisto et al., 2008; Somers, 2001) provide the basis for accomplishing everyday tasks (e.g., dressing, transferring in and out of bed, pressure relief, rolling over in bed). Individuals do not recover the ability to perform everyday tasks as performed prior to injury but are trained to accomplish tasks using a new behavioral strategy such as using an alternative body segment, an external aid, or physical assistance (Barbeau et al., 2006; Kleim, 2006). The reader is referred to the Spinal Cord Injury Rehabilitation Evidence, volume 2, for an up-to-date review of interventions (Chapter 7: Lower Limb Rehabilitation Following Spinal Cord Injury; http://www.scireproject.com/home.php).

Recovery of Posture and Walking After Stroke

Stroke is defined as a focal cerebrovascular event in which sudden loss of brain function caused by interruption of the flow of blood to the brain or by rupture of blood vessels in the brain persists beyond 24 hours. In the United States alone, over 795,000 individuals suffer a first-time or recurrent stroke annually (Lloyd-Jones et al., 2010). Stroke ranks as the seventh highest cause of burden of disease worldwide in terms of disability-adjusted life years and as the single most important cause of severe disability in people living at home (Lopez & Mathers, 2006). Of those who survive a stroke annually, 73% will incur subsequent disability. In 75% of the post-stroke population, walking dysfunction is a significant contributor to post-stroke disability and is associated with sensorimotor deficits and hemiparesis (Duncan, 2007).

Functional Deficits After Stroke

An impaired ability to walk is a significant contributor to long-term disability and burden of care after stroke. Approximately one third of people surviving acute stroke are unable to walk 3 months after admission to a general hospital (Wade et al., 1987). Those who do achieve independent walking are still limited in community ambulation, with motor impairments contributing to balance dysfunction post-stroke (Jorgensen et al., 1995). Individuals post-stroke with mild to moderate motor impairments who achieve ambulatory status are at significantly greater risk for falls (Forster & Young, 1995; Keenan et al., 1984). Of those who are ambulatory, 40% will have severe impairments including balance deficits, limiting ambulation to household status. With community ambulation, the risk of falls is 73% within 6 months after the stroke. The occurrence of a fall within this period compounds the risk for further fall incidence fourfold.

The gait pattern of individuals who have sustained a stroke was thoroughly described in a review by Olney and colleagues (1998). The two immediate impairments of most significance to gait performance are diminished strength, or the inability to generate voluntary muscle contractions of normal magnitude in any muscle groups, and inappropriately timed or inappropriately graded muscle activity. Reduced walking speed and longer stance phases have been observed for both the affected and unaffected lower limbs. Typically, the stance phase is longer in duration and occupies a greater proportion of the gait cycle on the unaffected side compared to the affected side. The third difference is a greater proportion of the gait cycle spent in double support in individuals post-stroke than that of able-bodied individuals walking at normal speeds. In addition, with hemiparesis, variations in joint excursions include several deviations at initial contact and reduced excursions during swing (Olney et al., 1998). Examples include decreased hip flexion at initial contact, increased hip flexion at toe-off, and decreased hip flexion during mid-swing; more knee flexion at initial contact and less knee flexion at toe-off and mid-swing; and more ankle plantarflexion at initial contact and mid-swing and less ankle plantarflexion at toe-off.

Studies have classified the kinematic patterns of individuals post-stroke into sub-groups (De Quervain et al., 1996; Sullivan et al., 2008) in combination with spatial temporal characteristics (Mulroy et al., 2003). Individuals with severe hemiparesis who walk slowly have been described by two kinematic patterns: extensor thrust or extended pattern and the buckling knee or flexed pattern. The extended pattern is characterized by increased ankle plantarflexion and knee hyperextension throughout the stance phase, with this pattern also dominating the flexor phase. Thus, insufficient ankle flexion and knee flexion are exhibited during swing. In contrast, the flexed pattern is characterized by increased ankle and knee flexion during stance with deficient hip extension prior to swing initiation. The walking kinematics of individuals with mild to moderate impairments and moderate to fast walking speeds are more comparable to those of healthy individuals. Moderate-speed walkers demonstrated a greater flexor pattern during stance (knee flexion) with decreased hip extension and plantarflexion at pre-swing compared to the faster walkers. Interestingly, the kinematics of the non-paretic leg also change after stroke. Such changes likely occur to compensate for the motor impairments of the paretic leg and may also reflect speed-dependent effects. Increased hip flexor moments were observed in late stance and were positively correlated to walking speed. Hip muscle activation may thus compensate for weak plantarflexors in some faster walkers post-stroke (Nadeau et al., 1999).

In comparison, when speeds are matched between post-stroke individuals and healthy controls, joint moment and power profiles are similar in pattern, yet differ in the amplitude (comparing hemiparetic to paretic legs and hemiparetic to healthy controls). Ankle joint plantarflexor power and moments are reduced or absent in the hemiparetic leg, in contrast to being equal or greater in the nonparetic legs. More recently, the anterior–posterior ground reaction force has been used to quantify the contribution of the paretic leg to forward propulsion during walking (Bowden et al., 2008). The percentage of paretic leg propulsion differs across stroke severity: severe (16%), moderate (36%), and mild hemiparesis (49% of normal). This measure may serve to discriminate between recovery or restitution of limb function and compensation after a therapeutic intervention (Sullivan et al., 2008).

Little is known about the contribution of the lower limbs and upper portions of the body to the adaptation of the gait pattern in post-stroke individuals. During normal gait, the main functions of the pelvis and trunk are to maintain body equilibrium and achieve smooth locomotion (Saunders et al., 2004; Thorstensson et al., 1984; Thurston & Harris, 1983; Wall et al., 1981). With gait pathologies such as stroke, movements of the pelvis and trunk may be used to compensate for lower limb deficits and show excessive range of motion.

Post-stroke individuals exhibit difficulties adapting their locomotor pattern to change speed and to uphill walking (Leroux et al., 1999). Unlike healthy subjects, who show a clear pattern of adaptation at the hip, knee, and ankle joints, post-stroke subjects mainly use the hip when adapting to uphill inclines. While the activation of plantarflexor muscles increases in control subjects during uphill walking, it does not in post-stroke subjects, a modification likely related to a weak push-off. Thus, a compensatory mechanism from axial and proximal muscles may be needed when adapting to inclined walking.

Furthermore, these compensatory mechanisms may depend on the severity of sensory or motor impairments. More impaired post-stroke individuals may use pelvis and trunk movements to a greater extent to compensate for lower limb deficits and adapt to different inclines. For instance, subjects with unilateral hip pain due to osteoarthritis (and avascular necrosis) use larger pelvic and trunk movements to compensate for limited hip motion (Thurston, 1985). These subjects show an abnormal lateral elevation of the pelvis during the swing phase to compensate for limited hip flexion and adopt a toe-floor clearance similar to normal walking. Excessive rotations from the pelvis and trunk have also been reported in subjects with hip pain (Thurston, 1985) and in those with hemiplegia due to stroke (Wagenaar & Beek, 1992). These studies show that abnormal movements from the trunk and pelvis can be used to overcome lower limb deficits in pathologic gait.

Physical Rehabilitation After Stroke

There are a number of different approaches to physical therapy following stroke. Prior to the 1940s, these primarily consisted of corrective exercises based on orthopaedic principles related to the contraction and relaxation of muscles, with emphasis placed on regaining function by compensating with the unaffected limbs (Langhorne et al., 1996). In the 1950s and 1960s, techniques based on available knowledge were developed, including the methods of Bobath (Davies, 1985; Lennon & Ashburn, 2000; Wagenaar & Beek, 1992) and Rood (Goff, 1969) and the proprioceptive neuromuscular facilitation approach (Knott, 1968). These approaches targeted activating weak muscles and reducing spasticity after stroke to normalize movements. In the 1980s, the potential importance of neuropsychology and motor learning (Schmidt & Lee, 2005) was understood and incorporated into post-stroke rehabilitation (Sullivan et al., 2008; Turnbull, 1982; Winstein et al., 2003, 2007). Recent evidence is mounting for effective rehabilitation of walking post-stroke that includes task-specific training, resisted strengthening for the upper and lower extremities, and aerobic training (Sullivan et al., 2008).

Alternatively, impairment-based strategies have also demonstrated benefits. Resisted strength training has predominantly been viewed as inappropriate in post-stroke persons due to concern for increased spasticity and abnormal movement patterns. However, evidence now indicates that strengthening can improve function without increased spasticity or greater dyscoordination (Foley et al., 2009). Similarly, aerobic training has addressed the effects of inactivity and resultant deconditioning post-stroke, particularly in the chronic condition. Because post-stroke individuals have a greater risk for a second stroke, exercise is highly recommended to decrease their risk. Specific guidelines and monitoring of vital signs allow aerobic exercise to be safely integrated into a rehabilitation program for post-stroke individuals, with benefits for cardiovascular health and walking. Various modes of training have been used, such as stationary cycling, treadmill walking, water-based exercise, overground walking, and stair climbing (Foley et al., 2009). The reader is referred to the Canadian Stroke Network for ongoing systematic review of the evidence for lower extremity training and mobility post-stroke.

Evidence-Based Practice

Physical rehabilitation is embarking on a new era requiring a paradigm shift in our thinking and clinical decision making. Neurorehabilitation, rather than relying primarily on traditional approaches based on the observation, skills, and assumptions from master clinicians (Adler et al., 1999; Bobath, 1979; Kleim, 2006; Knott, 1968), now emphasizes the important role of evidence-based medicine. *Evidence-based practice* is defined as a "conscientious, explicit and judicious use of best evidence in making decisions about individual patients" (Sackett, 1996). The practice of evidence-based medicine means integrating individual clinical expertise with the best available external clinical evidence from systematic research. Research evidence is one component of the clinical decision-making process and is combined with clinical expertise; client preferences, needs, and priorities; and available resources to result in the best practice and highest achievable level of recovery of function for each individual.

Implementing evidence-based practice requires accessing research findings, acquiring new knowledge, adopting new concepts, implementing new interventions, and performing objective evaluation. Academic programs in rehabilitation sciences led by multidisciplinary teams of researchers provide opportunities for the advancement of evidence-based neurorehabilitation practices for improving recovery for individuals after neurologic injury and disease.

The translation of evidence into practice is a new and challenging approach for physical therapists (Jette, 2006). The application of evidence-based therapy to today's academic programs, however, remains relatively new to many practitioners. In reviewing the evidence for a designated therapeutic intervention, it is important to distinguish the essential components that are different from other approaches. The evidence for much of neurorehabilitation practice is limited but has been disseminated in the clinical literature as summarized reviews of evidence and in the outcomes of such historical conferences such as NU-STEP (Northwestern University Special Therapeutic Exercise Project), II STEP, and III STEP (Callahan et al., 2006) to inform clinical decision making and practice.

Evidence-Based, Restorative Strategies for Rehabilitation After Neurologic Insult: Locomotor Training

New knowledge of the neurobiological control of walking and the plasticity of the nervous system in response to repetitive activity is reshaping the direction of physical rehabilitation after neurologic injury (Callahan et al., 2006). Partnerships of basic scientists, clinicians, and applied scientists, as exemplified in the authorship of this text, have resulted in translation of such knowledge from the laboratory to the human condition and formed the basis for activity-based therapies (Behrman & Harkema, 2008; Dromerick et al., 2006) such as Locomotor Training.

Several reviews of Locomotor Training provide detailed information and interpretations of the literature relative to clinical decision making and are recommended to the reader (Behrman et al., 2006; Lam et al., 2008; Mehrholz et al., 2008). In reviewing the literature, consideration should be given to the specific patient population, severity of injury, and time since injury. Not all neurologic patient populations will be represented in the literature, and some may actually never be tested within a randomized clinical trial or cohort studies because of their low prevalence in society. The good clinical judgment and expertise of the clinician, in combination with the literature, will allow for decision making to benefit subpopulations of clients with injury or disease. Publishing such case studies or case series may be very informative when gold standard randomized clinical trials examining large populations are not feasible and also may provide a valuable resource for clinicians implementing evidence-based practice.

In addition, when reviewing the evidence, the meaningfulness and relevance of outcome assessments for recovery of walking function should be considered carefully (Bowden et al., 2008; Lam et al., 2008; Mehrholz et al., 2008). For instance, while gait speed is an important outcome with functional relevance (Perry et al., 1995), change to a less restrictive assistive device (e.g., from a rolling walker to bilateral forearm crutches) may be accompanied by an initial decrease in gait speed or even an outcome with a slower gait speed, but it still indicates recovery. Even improvements in walking speed reported as large-percentage changes may not reflect meaningful changes in speed (e.g., a speed change from 0.03 m/s to 0.06 m/s is a 100% change) or result in functional walking recovery (Behrman & Harkema, 2007). Last, improvements in gait speed may be accomplished by a persistent and even enhanced compensated gait pattern (e.g., greater and faster hip hike and elevation to clear a foot during advancement of a limb as "swing") as opposed to neuromuscular recovery (i.e., a more upright trunk with increased hip extension and less upper extremity weight-bearing).

When reading the literature, clinicians will need to carefully review the methodology to understand the critical elements of the intervention and the variances among those presented. A case in point may best be seen by reviewing an article (Vidoni et al., 2008) reporting an intervention using a body weight support on the treadmill (BWST) that is accompanied by an online video of the intervention (http://www.jnptextra.org/pvideos. cfm#2; June 2008, video 1, BWST training, and September 2006, Video Limb Kinematics during Treadmill Walking). A quick review of this video noting "BWST" in the descriptors of the therapy will discern two very different approaches to a rehabilitation protocol with the aim of improving walking after stroke. While use of a BWST is a common denominator and the described interventions exhibit some similarity, the video representations of the training differ significantly from one another. Thus, the interventions, although noted as "BWST training," are not the same intervention. While the published visual aid for these two articles certainly provided clear differences, the reader of the literature more often is required to detect such differences from the written, published article alone. This remains a challenge but is a necessary step in conducting evidence-based practice. That said, the question remains as to what the active and critical ingredients in a therapy are as described in the literature. Such active ingredients may include the emphasis on specific and integrated afferent input (body weight load, treadmill speed, arm swing), manual- or robotic-assisted training, inclusion of overground training, duration and intensity of training, translation/integration beyond the clinic, and progression strategies.

In addition, while task-specific retraining is considered for stroke rehabilitation, clinical practice guidelines have not been specifically developed. Clearly identifying the active ingredients and exercise intensity of a therapeutic intervention will enhance the ability to assess and compare therapeutic interventions. While a recent Cochrane review (Moseley et al., 2005) concluded that there is inconclusive evidence that task-specific treadmill or body weight–supported treadmill training is effective after stroke, the heterogeneity of the population and variable training paradigms reported in the literature likely make comparisons difficult to interpret. Clinical efficacy and ongoing clinical trials

(Duncan, 2007, Pohl et al., 2002; Sullivan et al., 2002, 2007) should continue to pinpoint who will benefit relative to severity, when an intervention is beneficial relative to stroke onset, and training intensity (frequency and duration).

A further example of implementing evidence-based practice in the clinic is the Christopher and Dana Reeve Foundation NeuroRecovery Network (Harkema et al., 2011a b). The network, a set of seven clinical sites in the United States, has adopted Locomotor Training as a standardized activity-based therapy for rehabilitation of individuals with motor incomplete SCI. A standardized protocol is implemented and standardized outcomes are evaluated periodically throughout the intervention. This process allows for reassessment of the therapeutic program, its intensity and duration, and its effectiveness with specific populations and ultimately affords further knowledge that can be applied to clinical decision making. While the merit and benefit of activity-based therapies continue to be assessed in specific patient populations, the NeuroRecovery Network also addresses the challenges clinicians face to meet the therapeutic demands necessary to promote learning and behavioral change after neurologic injury. Evaluation of the outcomes from this unique programmatic venture into rehabilitation and healthcare for providing activity-based therapies will guide future clinical decision making for responders and non-responders and thus patient selection, selection of outcomes, and development of outcome measures to facilitate dissemination of new discoveries into everyday clinical practice.

References

Adler S, Beckers D, and Buck M (1999). PNF in Practice. Berlin: Springer.

Bajd T, Stefancic M, Matjacic Z, et al. (1997). Improvement in step clearance via calf muscle stimulation. Med Biol Eng Comput 35: 113–116.

Barbeau H, Nadeau S, and Garneau C (2006). Physical determinants, emerging concepts, and training approaches in gait of individuals with spinal cord injury. J Neurotrauma 23: 571–585.

Barbeau H, Norman K, Fung J, et al. (1998). Does neurorehabilitation play a role in the recovery of walking in neurological populations? Ann N Y Acad Sci 860: 377–392.

Barbeau H, Ladouceur M, Norman K, et al. (1999). Walking after spinal cord injury: evaluation, treatment, and functional recovery. Arch Phys Med Rehabil 80: 225–235.

Behrman AL, Bowden MG, and Nair PM (2006). Neuroplasticity after spinal cord injury and training: an emerging paradigm shift in rehabilitation and walking recovery. Phys Ther 86: 1406–1425.

Behrman AL and Harkema SJ (2007). Physical rehabilitation as an agent for recovery after spinal cord injury. Phys Med Rehabil Clin North Am 18: 183–202.

Behrman A, Druin E, Bowden M, and Harkema SJ (2009) Ambulation. In: Sisto SA, Druin E, Mach Sliwinski M (Eds.), Spinal Cord Injuries Management and Rehabilitation. St. Louis, MO: Mosby Elsevier, 380–399.

Blessey R (1978). Energy cost of normal walking. Orthop Clin North Am 9: 356–358.

Bobath B (1979). The application of physiological principles to stroke rehabilitation. Practitioner 223: 793–794.

Bogataj U, Gros N, Kljajic M, et al. (1995). The rehabilitation of gait in patients with hemiplegia: a comparison between conventional therapy and multichannel functional electrical stimulation therapy. Phys Ther 75: 490–502.

Boviatsis EJ, Kouyialis AT, Korfias S, et al. (2005). Functional outcome of intrathecal baclofen administration for severe spasticity. Clin Neurol Neurosurg 107: 289–295.

Bowden MG, Hannold EM, Nair PM, et al. (2008). Beyond gait speed: a case report of a multidimensional approach to locomotor rehabilitation outcomes in incomplete spinal cord injury. J Neurol Phys Ther 32: 129–138.

Brandell BR (1977). Functional roles of the calf and vastus muscles in locomotion. Am J Phys Med 56: 59–74.

Callahan J, Parlman K, Beninato M, et al. (2006). Perspective: impact of the IIISTEP conference on clinical practice. J Neurol Phys Ther 30: 157–166.

Cope TC, Bodine-Fowler SC, Fournier M, et al. (1986). Soleus motor units in chronic spinal transected cats: physiological and morphological alterations. J Neurophysiol 55(6): 1–19.

Davies P (1985). Steps to Follow: A Guide to the Treatment of Adult Hemiplegia. Berlin: Springer.

De Quervain IA, Simon SR, Leurgans S, et al. (1996). Gait pattern in the early recovery period after stroke. J Bone Joint Surg [Am] 78: 1506–1514.

Demirel G, Yilmaz H, Paker N, et al. (1998). Osteoporosis after spinal cord injury. Spinal Cord 36: 822–825.

Dietz V and Berger W (1983). Normal and impaired regulation of muscle stiffness in gait: a new hypothesis about muscle hypertonia. Exp Neurol 79: 680–687.

Dietz V, Quintern J, and Berger W (1981). Electrophysiological studies of gait in spasticity and rigidity. Evidence that altered mechanical properties of muscle contribute to hypertonia. Brain 104: 431–449.

Ditunno J and Scivoletto G (2009). Clinical relevance of gait research applied to clinical trials in spinal cord injury. Brain Res Bull 78: 35–42.

Dromerick AW, Lum PS, and Hidler J (2006). Activity-based therapies. NeuroRx 3: 428–438.

Duncan PW (2007). Barriers to evidence-based physical therapist practice for people after stroke: invited commentary. Phys Ther 83: 1304.

Foley N, Teasell R, and Bhogal S (2009). Mobility and the lower extremity. In: Evidence-Based Review of Stroke Rehabilitation (12th ed.). Canadian Stroke Network, 9: 1–128. Available at: http://www.ebrsr.com/uploads/Module_9_mobility.pdf

Forster A and Young J (1995). Incidence and consequences of falls due to stroke: a systematic inquiry. Br Med J 311: 83–86.

Fung J and Barbeau H (1994). Effects of conditioning musculo-cutaneous stimulation on the soleus H-reflex in normal and spastic subjects during walking and standing. J. Neurophysiol 72: 2090–2104.

Garland DE, Stewart CA, Adkins RH, et al. (1992). Osteoporosis after spinal cord injury. J Orthop Res 10: 371–378.

Gibson C, Turner S, and Donnelly M (2009). One Degree of Separation: Paralysis and Spinal Cord Injury in the United States. Short Hills, NJ: Christopher and Dana Reeve Foundation.

Go BK, DeVivo MJ, and Richards SJ (1995). The epidemiology of spinal cord injury. In: Stover SL, DeLisa JA, and Whiteneck GG (Eds.), Spinal Cord Injury: Clinical Outcomes from the Model Systems. Gaithersburg, MD: Aspen Publisher, Inc., 21–55.

Goff DW (1969). Spinal injury unit. Hospitals 43: 60–61.

Harkema SJ, Schmidt-Read, M, Behrman, AL, et al. (2011a). Establishing the NeuroRecovery Network: Multisite rehabilitation centers that provide activity-based therapies and assessments for neurologic disorders. Arch Phys Med Rehabil *In Press.*

Harkema SJ, Schmidt-Read, M, Lorenz DL, et al. (2011b). Balance and ambulation improvements in individuals with chronic incomplete spinal cord injury using Locomotor Training–based rehabilitation. Arch Phys Med Rehabil *In Press.*

Halstead LS and Grimby G (1995). Post-polio Syndrome. Philadelphia: Hanley and Belfus.

Hooker SP, Greenwood JD, Hatae DT, et al. (1993). Oxygen uptake and heart rate relationship in persons with spinal cord injury. Med Sci Sports Exerc 25: 1115–1119.

Hoy MG and Zernicke RF (1986). The role of intersegmental dynamics during rapid limb oscillations. J Biomech 19: 867–877.

Jette AM (2006). Toward a common language for function, disability, and health. Phys Ther 86: 726–734.

Jorgensen HS, Nakayama H, Raaschou HO, et al. (1995). Recovery of walking function in stroke patients: the Copenhagen Stroke Study. Arch Phys Med Rehabil 76: 27–32.

Keenan MA, Perry J, and Jordan C (1984). Factors affecting balance and ambulation following stroke. Clin Orthop Relat Res 165–171.

Kirshblum S (2004). New rehabilitation interventions in spinal cord injury. J Spinal Cord Med 27: 342–350.

Kleim JA (2006). III STEP: a basic scientist's perspective. Phys Ther 86: 614–617.

Knott LW (1968). Evaluation process in the rehabilitative program. Mod Treat 5: 893–899.

Krebs HI, Mernoff S, Fasoli SE, et al. (2008). A comparison of functional and impairment-based robotic training in severe to moderate chronic stroke: a pilot study. NeuroRehabilitation 23: 81–87.

Ladouceur M, Barbeau H, and McFadyen BJ (2003). Kinematic adaptations of spinal cord-injured subjects during obstructed walking. Neurorehabil Neural Repair 17: 25–31.

Lam T, Noonan VK, and Eng JJ (2008). A systematic review of functional ambulation outcome measures in spinal cord injury. Spinal Cord 46: 246–254.

Lange GW, Hintermeister RA, Schlegel T, et al. (1996). Electromyographic and kinematic analysis of graded treadmill walking and the implications for knee rehabilitation. J Orthop Sports Phys Ther 23: 294–301.

Langhorne P, Wagenaar R, and Partridge C (1996). Physiotherapy after stroke: more is better? Physiother Res Int 1: 75–88.

Lennon S and Ashburn A (2000). The Bobath concept in stroke rehabilitation: a focus group study of the experienced physiotherapists' perspective. Disabil Rehabil 22: 665–674.

Leroux A, Fung J, and Barbeau H (1999). Adaptation of the walking pattern to uphill walking in normal and spinal-cord injured subjects. Exp Brain Res 126: 359–368.

Leroux A, Fung J, and Barbeau H (2002). Postural adaptation to walking on inclined surfaces: I. Normal strategies. Gait Posture 15: 64–74.

Leroux A, Fung J, and Barbeau H (2006). Postural adaptation to walking on inclined surfaces: II. Strategies following spinal cord injury. Clin Neurophysiol 117: 1273–1282.

Lloyd-Jones D, Adams RJ, Brown TM, et al. (2010). Heart disease and stroke statistics 2010 update: a report from the American Heart Association. Circulation 121: e46–e215.

Lopez AD and Mathers CD (2006). Measuring the global burden of disease and epidemiological transitions: 2002–2030. Ann Trop Med Parasitol 100: 481–499.

Mehrholz J, Kugler J, and Pohl M (2008). Locomotor training for walking after spinal cord injury. Cochrane Database Syst Rev CD006676.

Melis EH, Torres-Moreno R, Barbeau H, et al. (1999). Analysis of assisted-gait characteristics in persons with incomplete spinal cord injury. Spinal Cord 37: 430–439.

Mirbagheri MM, Barbeau H, and Ladouceur M (2001). Intrinsic and reflex stiffness in normal and spastic spinal cord injured subjects. Exp Brain Res 141: 446–459.

Mirbagheri MM, Ladouceur M, Barbeau H, et al. (2002). The effects of long-term FES-assisted walking on intrinsic and reflex dynamic stiffness in spastic spinal-cord-injured subjects. IEEE Trans Neural Syst Rehabil Eng 10: 280–289.

Moseley AM, Stark A, Cameron ID, et al. (2005). Treadmill training and body weight support for walking after stroke. Cochrane Database Syst Rev CD002840.

Mulroy S, Gronley J, Weiss W, et al. (2003). Use of cluster analysis for gait pattern classification of patients in the early and late recovery phases following stroke. Gait Posture 18: 114–125.

Nadeau S, Arsenault AB, Gravel D, et al. (1999). Analysis of the clinical factors determining natural and maximal gait speeds in adults with a stroke. Am J Phys Med Rehabil 78: 123–130.

Noreau L and Shephard RJ (1995). Spinal cord injury, exercise and quality of life. Sports Med 20: 226–250.

Olney SJ, Griffin MP, and McBride ID (1998). Multivariate examination of data from gait analysis of persons with stroke. Phys Ther 78: 814–828.

Pepin A, Ladouceur M, and Barbeau H (2003a). Treadmill walking in incomplete spinal-cord-injured subjects: 2. Factors limiting the maximal speed. Spinal Cord 41: 271–279.

Pepin A, Norman KE, and Barbeau H (2003b). Treadmill walking in incomplete spinal-cord-injured subjects: 1. Adaptation to changes in speed. Spinal Cord 41: 257–270.

Perry J, Garrett M, Gromley J, et al. (1995). Classification of walking handicap in the stroke population. Stroke 26: 982–989.

Pohl M, Mehrholz J, Ritschel C, et al. (2002). Speed-dependent treadmill training in ambulatory hemiparetic stroke patients: a randomized controlled trial. Stroke 33: 553–558.

Quiben M (2006). The challenges of the late effects of polio: post-polio syndrome. In: Umphred D (Ed.), Neurological Rehabilitation (5th ed.). Elsevier, 940–957.

Raymond J, Davis GM, Fahey A, et al. (1997). Oxygen uptake and heart rate responses during arm vs. combined arm/electrically stimulated leg exercise in people with paraplegia. Spinal Cord 35: 680–685.

Sackett DL, Rosenberg WM, Gray JA, et al. (1996). Evidence-based medicine: what it is and what it isn't. Br Med J 312: 71–72.

Sadowsky CL and McDonald JW (2009). Activity-based restorative therapies: concepts and applications in spinal cord injury-related neurorehabilitation. Dev Disabil Res Rev 15: 112–116.

Saunders DH, Greig CA, Young A, et al. (2004). Physical fitness training for stroke patients. Cochrane Database Syst Rev CD003316.

Schmidt R and Lee T (2005). Motor Control and Motor Learning: A Behavioral Emphasis (4th ed.). Champaign, IL: Human Kinetics.

Schmidt R and Lee T (1999). Motor Control and Motor Learning: A Behavioral Emphasis (3rd ed.). Champaign, IL: Human Kinetics.

Sharrard W (1955). Muscle recovery in poliomyelitis. J Bone Joint Surg [Br] 37: 63–79.

Shumway-Cook A and Woollacott MH (1995). Motor Control: Theory and Practical Applications. Williams and Wilkins, Baltimore, MD.

Simonsen EB, Dyhre-Poulsen P, and Voigt M (1995). Excitability of the soleus H reflex during graded walking in humans. Acta Physiol Scand 153: 21–32.

Sinkjaer T, Andersen JB, and Larsen B (1996). Soleus stretch reflex modulation during gait in humans. J Neurophysiol 76: 1112–1120.

Sinkjaer T and Magnussen I (1994). Passive, intrinsic and reflex-mediated stiffness in the ankle extensors of hemiparetic patients. Brain 117(Pt 2): 355–363.

Sisto SA, Forrest GF, and Faghri PD (2008). Technology for mobility and quality of life in spinal cord injury. IEEE Eng Med Biol Mag 27: 56–68.

Somers M (2001). Spinal Cord Injury: Functional Rehabilitation. London: Prentice Hall Inc.

Stein RB, Gordon T, Jefferson J, et al. (1992). Optimal stimulation of paralyzed muscle after human spinal cord injury. J Appl Physiol 72: 1393–1400.

Stein RB, Yang J, Edamura M, et al. (1991). Reflex modulation during normal and pathological human locomotion. In: Shimamura M, Grillner S, and Edgerton VR (Eds.), Neurological Basis of Human Locomotion. Tokyo: Japan Scientific Societies Press, 335–346.

Stein RB, Yang JF, Belanger M, et al. (1993). Modification of reflexes in normal and abnormal movements. In: Allum JHJ, Allum-Mecklenburg D, Harris F, et al. (Eds.), Progress in Brain Research. Elsevier Science Publishers, 189–196.

Stover SL, DeVivo MJ, and Go BK (1999). History, implementation, and current status of the National Spinal Cord Injury Database. Arch Phys Med Rehabil 80: 1365–1371.

Sullivan K, Mulroy S, and Kautz S (2008). Walking recovery and rehabilitation after stroke. In: Stein J, Harvey RL, Macko RE, et al. (Eds.), Stroke Recovery and Rehabilitation. New York: Demos Medical Publishing.

Thilmann AF, Schwarz M, Topper R, et al. (1991). Different mechanisms underlie the long-latency stretch reflex response of active human muscle at different joints. J Physiol 444: 631–643.

Thorstensson A, Nilsson J, Carlson H, et al. (1984). Trunk movements in human locomotion. Acta Physiol Scand 121: 9–22.

Thurston AJ (1985). Spinal and pelvic kinematics in osteoarthrosis of the hip joint. Spine 10: 467–471.

Thurston AJ and Harris JD (1983). Normal kinematics of the lumbar spine and pelvis. Spine 8: 199–205.

Turnbull GI (1982). Some learning theory implications in neurological physiotherapy. Physiotherapy 68: 38–41.

Veltink PH, Ladouceur M, and Sinkjaer T (2000). Inhibition of the triceps surae stretch reflex by stimulation of the deep peroneal nerve in persons with spastic stroke. Arch Phys Med Rehabil 81: 1016–1024.

Vidoni ED, Tull A, and Kluding P (2008). Use of three gait-training strategies in an individual with multiple, chronic strokes. J Neurol Phys Ther 32: 88–96.

Wade DT, Wood VA, Heller A, et al. (1987). Walking after stroke. Measurement and recovery over the first 3 months. Scand J Rehabil Med 19: 25–30.

Wagenaar RC and Beek WJ (1992). Hemiplegic gait: a kinematic analysis using walking speed as a basis. J Biomech 25: 1007–1015.

Wall JC, Nottrodt JW, and Charteris J (1981). The effects of uphill and downhill walking on pelvic oscillations in the transverse plane. Ergonomics 24: 807–816.

Whiteneck G, Gassaway J, Dijkers M, et al. (2009). New approach to study the contents and outcomes of spinal cord injury rehabilitation: the SCIRehab Project. J Spinal Cord Med 32: 251–259.

Wilmet E, Ismail AA, Heilporn A, et al. (1995). Longitudinal study of the bone mineral content and of soft tissue composition after spinal cord section. Paraplegia 33: 674–677.

Winstein C, Pate P, Ge T, et al. (2008). The Physical Therapy Clinical Research Network (PTClinResNet): methods, efficacy, and benefits of a rehabilitation research network. Am J Phys Med Rehabil 87: 937–950.

Winstein CJ, Miller JP, Blanton S, et al. (2003). Methods for a multisite randomized trial to investigate the effect of constraint-induced movement therapy in improving upper extremity function among adults recovering from a cerebrovascular stroke. Neurorehabil Neural Repair 17: 137–152.

Wisleder D, Zernicke RF, and Smith JL (1990). Speed-related changes in hindlimb intersegmental dynamics during the swing phase of cat locomotion. Exp Brain Res 79: 651–660.

Yamamoto M, Tajima F, Okawa H, et al. (1999). Static exercise-induced increase in blood pressure in individuals with cervical spinal cord injury. Arch Phys Med Rehabil 80: 288–293.

Yang J, Stein RB, Jhamandas J, et al. (1990). Motor unit numbers and contractile properties after spinal cord injury. Ann Neurol 28: 496–502.

Yang JF, Fung J, Edamura M, et al. (1991). H-reflex modulation during walking in spastic paretic subjects. Can J Neurol Sci 18: 443–452.

2

Evidence for Locomotor Training

Chapter Outline

Chapter Objectives

The objectives of Chapter 2 are to:

1. Understand the scientific and clinical evidence underlying Locomotor Training.
2. Define *activity-dependent plasticity*.

3. Define *task-specific training*.
4. List the principles of Locomotor Training.
5. Describe the role of sensory input in generating locomotion in animals and humans.

Summary

Locomotor Training is an emerging rehabilitation intervention for recovery of function after neurologic injury or disease, and the physiologic basis and scientific evidence supporting its use will be presented in this chapter. As an activity-based therapy, Locomotor Training provides activation of the neuromuscular system below the level of the lesion, with the goal of retraining the nervous system to recover specific motor tasks related to mobility, posture, standing, and walking. Locomotor Training principles have emerged from results of basic science studies in animals and humans that will be discussed in this chapter.

Neural Control of Locomotion

The loss of standing and walking in humans after neurologic injury or disease has been primarily attributed to the dominance of supraspinal over spinal mechanisms in the control of locomotion (Dietz et al., 1992; Fouad & Pearson, 2004; Kuhn, 1950; Mulroy et al., 2003; Nadeau et al., 1999; Vilensky & O'Connor, 1997). Descending supraspinal input has been considered as primarily responsible for the activation of the lower limb motor neurons in humans, and consequently, after neurologic injury or disease, the prognosis for recovery of walking is estimated from the movements that individuals can generate in isolated muscle groups of the limbs (Burns et al., 1997; Crozier et al., 1992; Hussey & Stauffer, 1973; Mulroy et al., 2003; Waters et al., 1993, 1994). Thus, the role of the spinal cord and the importance of afferent input in generating successful human locomotion (Dietz, 1987; Duysens et al., 1998, 2000) has been considered unimportant after the loss of supraspinal input. However, the predominant role of spinal neural circuitry interacting with afferent input in control of locomotion is well accepted in essentially all other nonhuman species, and the evidence is summarized below.

Central Pattern Generation

Central pattern generation describes the mechanisms of the neural networks of the lumbosacral spinal cord that interact with supraspinal, propriospinal, and afferent input to generate successful locomotion (Grillner, 1981; Jankowska, 1992; McCrea, 2001; Pearson, 2004; Sherrington, 1900). Specific properties of these spinal interneuronal networks and their interaction with afferent input are critical for locomotion. Spinal cord neuronal networks have the capacity to activate an oscillatory motor pattern similar to locomotion even without input from supraspinal centers or the periphery. In addition, these networks are functionally organized so that flexor and extensor motor pools influence each other and can modulate interlimb coordination. Finally, the interaction of these spinal interneurons with specific afferent input generated by specific sensory cues related to standing and stepping is essential for successful locomotion.

The details of the general anatomic location and the neurophysiologic properties of these spinal interneurons have been studied in species from cockroaches, to lamprey, to mammals (Grillner, 1981; Jankowska & Riddell, 1995). In this chapter we will not discuss these specific details but rather will focus on the neuronal mechanisms that support the interaction of these spinal networks with afferent and supraspinal input that is important for successful locomotion. These properties have not been recognized historically in neurorehabilitation and thus have not been extensively used in rehabilitative strategies for recovery of function after neurologic injury and disease in humans.

Interaction of Sensory Input with Spinal Cord Interneuronal Networks

Understanding the interactions of sensory input and spinal networks during standing and stepping led to several landmark studies that demonstrated successful stepping in mammals could occur in the absence of supraspinal influence (Barbeau & Rossignol, 1987; de Guzman et al., 1991; de Leon et al., 1999b; Forssberg, 1979a; Forssberg et al., 1977, 1980; Lovely et al., 1986, 1990; Rossignol et al., 1986). Early studies demonstrated that interlimb coordination and the velocity of stepping were controlled by the spinal cord, as kittens that had a transected spinal cord were able to step on a treadmill (Forssberg et al., 1980). The importance of sensory information during stepping was shown by the ability of these kittens to adjust to changes in treadmill speed and obstacles (Forssberg, 1979b) and to react to mechanical stimulation differently depending on the phase of the step cycle (Forssberg et al., 1977). The motor response to touching the dorsum of the paw during swing resulted in a flexion movement, while stimulation during stance did not. Electrical stimulation showed similar results indicating the spinal neural networks are capable of integrating complex sensory information to produce the most appropriate motor output for the current task in a phase-dependent manner (Forssberg, 1979a).

At first it was considered that only developing nervous systems had this capacity without supraspinal influence. However, in the 1980s this capacity was then shown in adult cats that regained the ability to walk with their hindlimbs on a treadmill after a complete transection (Barbeau & Rossignol, 1987; de Guzman et al., 1991). After spinalization, when properly trained, cats eventually regained plantar foot contact and weight support of the hindquarters (Rossignol et al., 1986). They were observed to walk up to 1.2 m/s on the treadmill with reciprocal alternation between the two hindlimbs. Increasing the treadmill speed resulted in a shortening of the stance phase, while the swing phase remained relatively constant. The hindlimb movements and motor patterns during walking after spinalization were surprisingly similar when comparing the behavior before spinalization in the same cat (Belanger et al., 1996). The loss of supraspinal control of gait resulted in deficiencies in goal-directed walking and balance requiring continual manual guidance to prevent falling. However, following a complete thoracic spinal cord transection, adult cats also could regain overground walking ability when a harness was used to compensate for the loss of balance control (Rossignol et al., 1986). When moving forward, the forelimbs induced the hindlimbs to move, and appropriate intralimb and interlimb coordination, dictated by forelimb movement, was observed.

Activity-Dependent Plasticity and Task-Specific Training

The specific training critical to this recovery of stepping was task-specific and reliant on the appropriate sensory cues related to the defined motor task. For example, it was shown specifically that hip position and unloading of the contralateral limb in combination initiates the swing phase movement (Grillner & Rossignol, 1978). Hip position is critical to this adjustment, and preventing extension can prevent the transition from flexor to extensor activity. Further evidence of the necessity of task-specific training was the observation that animals with complete transection of the spinal cord that were trained to walk or stand attained a very different level of performance (de Leon et al., 1998a, 1998b, 1999a, 1999b, 1999c). Animals that were trained to walk achieved a faster walking speed and more successful steps than animals that were trained only to stand. Similarly, animals that were trained to stand performed better standing than animals who were not trained.

In spinal cats, this capacity for adaptation was achieved via intense locomotor training alone or in combination with pharmacologic approaches such as the noradrenergic agonist clonidine (Chau et al., 1998, Edgerton et al., 1992). Six days of daily training plus pharmacologic treatment resulted in marked acceleration and improvement of the hindlimb walking pattern compared with the 2 to 3 weeks required to see such improvements with training alone. Further, complete spinal cats trained to walk at higher speeds performed better, suggesting that behavioral plasticity occurs within the spinal cord (Barbeau & Rossignol, 1987).

Further evidence of spinal plasticity was shown when spinal cats adapted to peripheral deficits from selected neuroectomies by training (Bouyer et al., 2001; Bouyer & Rossignol, 1998; Carrier et al., 1997; Rossignol et. al 1996; Rossignol et al., 2002). For example, surgical section of all cutaneous nerves of the foot below the ankle of cats caused a major deficit when walking on a horizontal ladder, but they recovered treadmill locomotion within a few days. However, after spinalization, the cats were unable to even place their feet on the belt. This suggests that although the animals may have the ability to compensate for the missing cutaneous information by other sensory cues, the spinal cord must be intact for the animals to walk properly with plantar foot contact. These findings suggested that some process of plasticity occurs within the spinal cord as a result of the locomotor adaptation even without supraspinal control.

These studies spanning over five decades elucidated the incredible level of control the spinal neural circuitry has in generating locomotion when driven by essential task-specific sensory cues. Interestingly, throughout the majority of time these studies were published there was an ongoing clear skepticism by scientists and clinicians that these mechanisms could play an important role in human locomotion. However, in the past 30 years, evidence from humans has indicated that many similar mechanisms as described here can also be attributed to the human spinal cord.

Evidence of Sensory Processing by Human Spinal Networks

The evidence for central pattern generation in humans is limited due to the inability to conclusively isolate the circuitry from descending and afferent input (Bussel et al., 1989, 1996; Calancie et al., 1994; Dimitrijevic et al., 1998; Gerasimenko et al., 2002).

Consequently, the question of whether the same relationships exist between sensory input and the spinal networks in humans after spinal cord injury (SCI) has been the catalyst for important translational research. The experimental paradigm has focused on the human spinal cord's capacity to generate locomotor patterns in the absence of supraspinal input, the interdependence of extensor and flexor motor pools, and the capacity for interlimb coordination (Dietz & Harkema 2004; Harkema, 2008).

Studies were conducted in both infants and adults as done in the animal studies. Yang and colleagues showed that infants as young as 10 days old could step on a treadmill and would adjust their locomotor pattern according to the speed of the belt, suggesting that the spinal cord can generate locomotor behavior in the absence of appropriate supraspinal input (or early in development) (Yang et al., 1998).

In addition, the functional capacity of the adult human spinal circuitry to interact with sensory input during locomotion was studied with individuals who have a functionally or clinically complete SCI. Individuals were characterized as clinically complete when they are classified using the American Spinal Injury Association Impairment Scale (AIS; Marino et al., 2003) as A, with no sensory or motor function detectable below the level of lesion and with no response with testing of lower leg sensory evoked potentials (Curt & Dietz, 1999). In humans with clinically complete SCI, motor patterns are observed during manually facilitated stepping on a treadmill with partial body weight support (BWS), indicating the capacity of the spinal cord to generate locomotor-like patterns (Beres-Jones & Harkema, 2004; Dietz et al., 1994, 1995; 1998; Dietz & Colombo, 2004, Dietz & Harkema 2004; Dobkin et al., 1995; Harkema et al., 1997). The motor output (EMG), in this case, must be driven by the sensory information available to the interneuronal networks of the spinal cord. The intrinsic neuronal organization of these networks was further understood by studying the relationship of efferent output among flexors and extensors and the response to task-specific practice.

Sensory input provides critical information to generate locomotor-like output by the functionally isolated human spinal cord (Beres-Jones et al., 2003; Beres-Jones & Harkema, 2004; Dietz et al., 1994; Dietz and Harkema, 2004; Ferris et al., 2004; Harkema, 2008; Harkema et al., 1997; Maegele et al., 2002, Sinkjaer et al., 1996). In individuals with clinically incomplete and complete SCI, stepping results in improved motor recruitment and reciprocity between agonists and antagonists compared with voluntary efforts intended to produce similar movements of flexion and extension of the hip, knee, and ankle (Maegele et al., 2002). Alternation of ankle flexors and extensors can occur, even in individuals with clinically complete SCI, indicating that the segmental influence of spinal networks can play a significant role in appropriate functional organization of motor output (Harkema, 2008).

The level of loading during stepping provides specific afferent cues that result in significant increases in the amplitude of motor pool activity of extensors and flexors independent of the level of supraspinal input available to the spinal networks (Dietz, 1998; Dietz et al., 2002; Harkema et al., 1997; Kojima et al., 1999). Even weight-bearing without movement of one leg can elicit rhythmic EMG activity during unilateral stepping (Ferris et al., 2004). Temporal and spatial distribution of load-related input also plays an important role in the generation of motor patterns during stepping when supraspinal input is limited (Beres-Jones & Harkema, 2004). Velocity-dependent modulation of locomotor patterns was observed in individuals without detectable supraspinal input available to spinal networks. The rate at which afferent input is delivered to the central nervous system may be important in more complex regulation of efferent patterns.

The human spinal networks also have the capacity to modulate interlimb coordination (Ferris et al., 2004). The human spinal networks can use sensory information about contralateral leg movements and loading to increase muscle activation even when there is no limb movement. Movement and loading in one limb can produce rhythmic muscle activity in the other limb even when it is stationary and unloaded in individuals with clinically complete SCI. Load-related information in the contralateral leg is necessary to produce these rhythmic patterns. Interestingly, when infants were stepped on a split-belt treadmill, each leg stepped according to the speed and direction of its belt, suggesting that the pattern generator for each limb is autonomous, but because the relationship between the legs remained reciprocal (so that swing occurred in only one leg at a time), the implication is that these separate networks interact with and influence one another (Yang et al., 2005).

The relative amplitude of EMG activity is lower in individuals with complete SCI compared with individuals with incomplete SCI and non-disabled individuals and may be a result of the level of activation of remaining supraspinal pathways on the spinal networks. The motor pattern variability is likely influenced by the time since injury, extent of ongoing neuromuscular activity below the lesion, the history of antispasticity and other medication use (Dietz et al., 1997), as well as other factors that remain undetermined. In addition, the possibility of residual supraspinal input available to the spinal networks that cannot be detected by routine clinical measures may influence the motor output (Sherwood et al., 1992). The observation that the functionally isolated human spinal cord has the capacity to generate locomotor patterns demonstrates that afferent feedback related to locomotion is sufficient to produce oscillatory, rhythmic, alternating efferent output related to the phases of the step cycle. This knowledge can be used to retrain the nervous system for standing and walking after neurologic injury.

Translation of Scientific Evidence into a Rehabilitation Intervention

Traditionally, rehabilitation has focused on functional recovery only when there was evidence of some voluntary control of the muscles needed for the task. This approach has been challenged by the findings of basic scientists studying the control of walking and activity-dependent plasticity that occurs in the human spinal cord. Their work has become the foundation for physiologically based approaches to enhance recovery after neurologic insult via physical rehabilitation and task-specific activity, practice, repetition, and challenge (Edgerton et al., 1991).

Activity-Based Therapy (Locomotor Training)

The neurophysiologic mechanisms described above have been translated into an evolving activity-based rehabilitation therapy for mobility, posture, standing, and walking. Locomotor Training, as described in this book, is based on scientific evidence and focuses on retraining the injured nervous system by driving neural plasticity by task-specific training (Harkema, 2001). This retraining is primarily driven by providing the needed sensory cues to the spinal cord circuitry. In cases of incomplete SCI and stroke, the entire neuroaxis is available for retraining and the residual supraspinal input is integrated for functional recovery. The knowledge from the scientific and clinical studies is transformed into guiding principles to provide a framework for clinical decision making, as well as a reference point for evaluating the potential application of any new modality, equipment, or therapeutic component.

The ensemble of sensory information during retraining is important in providing a clear picture of the task of walking to be synthesized and integrated by the nervous system to generate an effective motor response. The specific information being supplied is to be consistent with the movements and posture that are identified with the task of walking. As much as possible, the training should "train like you walk." The sensorimotor experience of Locomotor Training approximates the task of walking with increasing demands or challenges placed on the nervous system to adapt. Four guiding principles can be applied in any environment (clinic, home, or community) and provide a framework for decision making and choices that promote recovery of function.

Maximize Weight-Bearing on the Legs (Principle 1)

This principle can be accomplished by maximizing load-bearing of the lower extremities and minimizing load-bearing by the upper extremities. Increases in lower limb EMG amplitude are associated with increased load-bearing in animals and humans after SCI, as well as able-bodied individuals (Finch et. al 1991; Harkema et al., 1997). This physiological response to the sensory input associated with load-bearing translated into a guiding principle provides the opportunity to improve activation in muscles that, under voluntary conditions (i.e., manual muscle testing), are weak or do not produce a contraction (Maegele et al., 2002). Animal and human studies suggest that appropriate loading (loading and unloading) is very important (Dietz, 2001; Pearson, 2004). In fact, there is increasing evidence that during locomotion, afferent inputs from the ankle extensors lead to autogenic excitation rather than inhibition. The mechanism of the effect is still unclear, but recent studies strongly support the role of modulation of extensor load receptors probably arising from Golgi tendon organs (Pearson, 2004).

Visintin and Barbeau observed that shared load-bearing between the upper and lower limbs diminished EMG activity in the lower limbs (Visintin & Barbeau, 1989). In contrast, providing partial BWS through vertical suspension produced a relative increase in lower limb EMG activity and better timing between flexor and extensor muscle activation. Thus, minimizing upper limb loading during retraining by use of handrails or parallel bars is discouraged and increasing vertical load-bearing through the legs is encouraged. Furthermore, overground, the choice of an assistive device or gait pattern with a device may be made to reinforce lower limb loading versus upper limb weight-bearing.

Finally, appropriate loading during the support phase not only enhances ipsilateral extensor activity and increases the vertical force during the support phase but also triggers the swing phase in the contralateral limb (Dietz, 1996). Thus, interlimb coordination is functionally incorporated in the Locomotor Training paradigm to promote extensor activity in one limb and flexor activity in the contralateral limb. This represents a newly discovered function for these receptors in the regulation of different phases of walking in the SCI population (Dietz et al., 2002).

Optimize Sensory Cues (Principle 2)

Normal walking speed for an adult ranges approximately from 1.0 to 1.5 m/s (2.2 to 3.5 mph) and affords the spatial-temporal sequence of inputs that contribute to the characteristic sensorimotor experience of walking. Beres-Jones and Harkema (2004) and Lunenburger et al. (2006) observed velocity-dependent modulation of EMG activity in persons with both incomplete and complete SCI and in able-bodied individuals. Again, in an effort to increase muscle activation, the higher speeds may provide a stronger stimulus-response.

The important role of sensory inputs has been shown in several animal studies. First, Forssberg (1979b) provided evidence indicating that afferent inputs during hip extension are very important in resetting and entraining the locomotor rhythm (see Rossignol et al. [2006] for comprehensive review). Second, the modulation of reflexes has been shown to be task- and phase-specific in intact and spinalized cats as well as in human subjects (Duysens et al., 1990; Yang et al., 1991). For example, mechanical or electrical stimulation of the paw or of the cutaneous nerve during the flexor activity produces an increase in ipsilateral flexor EMG as well as the contralateral extensor EMG, but when the stimulus is delivered during the ipsilateral extensor muscle activity, it increases extensor muscle activity (Rossignol, 2000).

Duysens and coworkers (1990) and Zehr and colleagues (1997) have shown that cutaneous feedback from the foot is also especially important in human locomotion. They observed that reflex responses are particularly important in reactions to unexpected perturbations. The use of footwear with light soles during training on the treadmill or even overground can provide greater cutaneous input and is, thus, favored.

Sensory inputs may be necessary to stimulate the locomotor pattern not only for specific controls (step length, foot placement) but also as a crucial sensory input provided during the recovery process following a central nervous system insult (Duysens et al., 2004). Speed as a critical training variable and sensory cue has been tested in several clinical studies in post-stroke individuals. Training that occurs at faster walking speeds than can be achieved overground and approaches normal walking speeds results in better locomotor outcomes (Pohl et al., 2002; Sullivan et al., 2002).

Optimize the Kinematics (i.e., Trunk, Pelvis, and Lower Extremities) for Each Motor Task (Principle 3)

One kinematic component that is critical to successful walking is the transition from stance to swing. This transition may be neurally activated by the sensory input associated with hip extension (relative to an upright trunk) and limb load-bearing (muscle/tendon stretch, proprioception, cutaneous input), followed by unloading of the limb while transferring weight to the other limb. These two sensory elements, extension and load, are part of the essential ensemble of afferent input affording the transition and generation of activity from stance to swing or extension to flexion. Incorporating these elements into the training regimen is critical to initiating and generating flexion in the gait cycle. As the arms typically swing in reciprocal coordination with the lower limbs while walking, this automatic pattern and kinematic component may be of benefit in achieving a more complete sensory experience of walking. Furthermore, arm-swing may contribute to activity-dependent plasticity and development of appropriate balance responses and is thus encouraged by the trainer as opposed to a supportive function by the upper extremities.

The premise that sensory input is critical to retraining the nervous systems (Dietz & Harkema 2004; Harkema 2001) indicates that all joints movements (pelvis/hip, knee, and ankle) during the intervention should reflect those that occurred prior to injury for the specific motor task.

Maximize Recovery Strategies; Minimize Compensation Strategies (Principle 4)

Recovery strategies promote use of the inherent properties of the nervous system to generate motor responses within the usual kinematic framework. For instance, Visintin and Barbeau (1989) concluded that using parallel bars for upper extremity support produces a forward-flexed trunk, asymmetry in gait, and use of compensatory strategies for swing initiation such as "hip-hiking" (e.g., the trunk flexes laterally while raising the hip and advancing the leg forward with the knee extended). By comparison, vertical support provides a more upright trunk, hip extension and loading promoting the transition from stance to swing, and relatively fewer compensatory movement strategies while walking and would be more consistent with the Locomotor Training principles. Throughout retraining, individuals are encouraged to attempt movements but are assisted, as needed, to perform them to achieve the relevant task-specific sensory experience. Compensation also is likely to limit recovery as the sensory cues associated with the task will be very different or absence resulting in a neural plasticity that is not consistent with recovery of the function.

Clinical Evidence for Functional Recovery in Spinal Cord Injury

In humans with neurologic diseases, modern concepts of motor learning favor a task-specific repetitive approach to rehabilitation (Asanuma & Pavlides, 1997; Barbeau et al., 1993). For example, several studies found a decrease in spasticity when the spastic ankle is fixed in dorsiflexion by use of a tilt table, cast, or ankle–foot orthosis, but no change in the walking velocity and performance could be observed. Interestingly, nonspecific rehabilitation approaches such as passive stretching (Tremblay et al., 1990), acupuncture, transcutaneous electrical nerve stimulation (Johansson et al., 2001), or general home exercise have had no beneficial effects on functional locomotor outcomes.

Evidence indicates that Locomotor Training can be more effective than treatment using more traditional concepts (Behrman et al., 2005; Behrman & Harkema, 2000; Wernig et al., 1995; Wernig & Müller, 1992; Wirz et al., 2001). Task-specific therapeutic approaches contrast markedly with rehabilitation approaches that focus on decreasing spasticity or are nonspecific. One of the earliest clinical studies showed a major effect of Locomotor Training in chronic incomplete SCI individuals (Wernig & Müller, 1992). In another study in individuals with acute and chronic incomplete SCI, step training using body weight support on the treadmill (BWST) was superior to conventional physiotherapy for restoring walking and improving overground walking speed (Wernig et al., 1995). In a randomized clinical trial of individuals with ASIA C and D within 51 days of SCI, the effects of step training with BWS was exceptional at 6-month follow-up (>1.0 m/s mean walking speed) but not superior to the control group that had been trained overground at the same intensity of weight-bearing. Stratification of subjects in the BWST group by initial walking speed demonstrated an increased rate of recovery three times higher in individuals with incomplete SCI with an initial speed less than 0.3 m/s and two times higher with subjects walking initially greater than 0.6 m/s. For subjects walking between greater than 0.6 m/s and less than 1.2 m/s, no statistical difference was observed.

Locomotor Training may also improve walking speed in the chronic stages of injury. This has been suggested by studies of individuals with incomplete SCI, but the magnitude of change is less than that seen in the subacute stages (Barbeau et al., 1998a, 1998b; Gorassini, 2009). Preliminary results from trials using Locomotor Training combined with functional electrical stimulation and/or pharmacologic approaches showed great potential for individuals with chronic incomplete SCI (Ditunno & Scivoletto, 2009).

The population with motor incomplete SCI has demonstrated the greatest gains from Locomotor Training, whether provided during the acute rehabilitation phase (up to 12 months after injury) or greater than 12 months after injury (Behrman et al., 2005; Behrman & Harkema, 2000; Dietz, 2009; Gorassini et al., 2009; Harkema et al., 2010; Hicks et al., 2005, Wernig et al., 1995; Wernig & Müller, 1992; Wirz et al., 2001). Clinically meaningful improvements are reported for gait speed, endurance (distance ambulated), independence, locomotor adaptability, and classification of walking ability. The earlier the intervention is provided (less than 4 weeks after SCI), the faster the walking speed and the greater the distance achieved (Dobkin et al., 2006). This is seen particularly in subjects who changed AIS classifications within 4 and 6 weeks after injury (e.g., B to C or C to D) and thus in persons beginning therapy at a lower level of motor function.

While conventional overground training during the subacute phase of rehabilitation after motor incomplete SCI compared with Locomotor Training in a randomized clinical trial resulted in comparable and surprisingly significant outcomes in gait speed 6 and 12 months after SCI, all subjects received 60 minutes of weight-bearing and 60 sessions of therapy (Dobkin et al., 2006). Both of these factors may have contributed to the remarkable gait speeds achieved by both groups (mean gait speed 1.0 m/s); such intensity and duration may have been important factors not usually provided in current rehabilitation practice. Both of these factors, load and intensity, thus continue to serve as key guidelines for providing training regardless of the modality or environment. Whether extended duration would have had greater impact on walking recovery is not known; this typically is a variable that is limited in the design of large randomized clinical trials.

Locomotor Training in the population with chronic motor incomplete SCI has resulted in functional improvements in gait as well (Harkema et al., 2011). In a chronic population of individuals with incomplete SCI (AIS C and D), 89% significantly improved balance and ambulation. The greater the time since injury, the greater the period of locomotor training required to produce meaningful changes (Barbeau et al., 1998a, 1998b). This outcome may be due to the persistence of compensatory strategies (Barbeau et al., 2006) developed as one body part or system substituted for another to afford ambulation. Retraining thus involves the undoing of a habit and the learning of a new pattern of activation for successful walking.

Incorporating walking speed and postural demands into locomotor interventions is essential to the process of retraining walking. Continued adaptations during training will decrease energy cost (Ladouceur & Barbeau, 2000a, 2000b), decrease use of walking aids, and improve the ability to adapt the locomotor pattern and posture to uphill and downhill slopes and obstacles. Training at a comfortable speed will not challenge locomotor performance (unpublished results) as much as will challenging the speed of walking during training. Thus, to improve locomotor and postural adaptation, it is important, first, to understand the limiting control mechanisms and, second, to identify important determinant variables that could be used to evaluate proper challenge to locomotion and posture and to incorporate them into a training strategy.

The use of the Locomotor Training modality in individuals with complete SCI or with sensory sparing alone has not produced gains in walking ability to date. For this population, the benefits of Locomotor Training may be as exercise that reduces the secondary complications of SCI (e.g., bone loss, muscle atrophy, impaired circulation and pressure sores, weight gain, diabetes) and improves quality of life (Forrest et al., 2008; Hannold et al., 2006; Harkema et al., 2008; Jayaraman et al., 2008; Phillips et al., 2004) all which are critically important to those with SCI (Anderson 2004).

Clinical Evidence for Functional Recovery in Stroke

Recent systematic reviews indicate that organized (stroke unit) care decreases physical dependence after stroke compared with general medical care. This medical care is characterized by early mobilization and a multidisciplinary team. Walking on a treadmill with partial BWS is a method of improving walking after stroke that is becoming increasingly popular. This intervention permits a greater number of steps to be performed (task repetition) within a training session; thus, it increases the amount of task-specific practice completed. For example, Hesse and colleagues (1994) reported that a post-stroke individual can perform up to 1,000 steps in a 20-minute step training session on a treadmill, compared with only 50 to 100 steps during a 20-minute session of conventional physiotherapy. The speed of the treadmill, the amount of BWS, and the amount of assistance provide a sufficient training intensity. Since then, training with partial BWS has been increasingly promoted as a treatment to drive recovery after stroke (Hesse et al., 1995, 1997, 1999; Shepherd & Carr, 1999).

Another important piece of evidence of the effects of task-specific training is the finding that training while standing could improve balance but not gait after stroke (Winstein et al., 1989). Winstein and colleagues observed an improvement in balance during standing when post-stroke individuals had been trained to shift weight onto the hemiparetic side and bear weight symmetrically. However, the improvement in symmetry during standing did not transfer to walking, again suggesting the importance of task-specific training. In another study, Dean and collaborators (2007) trained post-stroke individuals to improve sitting balance symmetry. Although sitting symmetry did improve, symmetry during standing did not change, nor did it carry over to walking. Such studies explain, in part, why neurologic patients who have been trained with conventional rehabilitation approaches demonstrate minimal improvements in walking speed and in walking symmetry (Barbeau et al., 1999).

Results of a randomized clinical trial study indicated that post-stroke individuals with an initial walking speed less than 0.3 m/s demonstrated the greatest improvements at 6-month follow-up to Locomotor Training (Visintin et al., 1998). Other studies showed positive results with manually facilitated Locomotor Training post-stroke (Hornby et al., 2008, Roopchand et al., 2005). A recent Cochrane review (Moseley et al., 2005) on the use of treadmill training and BWS for walking rehabilitation after stroke

(15 clinical trials; 622 participants) found that the evidence was inconclusive to determine effectiveness for improving walking after stroke. However, the Cochrane review states that the evidence for training effectiveness is most conclusive in persons with mild gait impairment post-stroke.

Depending on the severity of the patient's injury and the time since the injury, recovery of walking may be achieved by applying challenging, task-specific approaches. Several clinical trials demonstrated major improvements in walking speed and functional recovery. In fact, individuals with incomplete SCI and those post-stroke with a low functional level (<0.4 m/s initial gait speed) benefit from locomotor training using the BWST to challenge both the posture and the walking speed (Kosak & Reding, 2000; Lewek et al., 2009; Visintin & Barbeau, 1989). Individuals with incomplete SCI and post-stroke with initial walking speeds of 0.4 m/s and above (Nilsson et al., 2001) benefit from a combination of locomotor training using BWST and overground training to challenge both walking speed and balance. Challenging walking and balance should be an important prerequisite for fundamental and clinical changes, but challenges should also be graded according to the severity of the patient's functional limitations (Duncan, 2007).

Evidence summarized in this chapter demonstrates the great potential for locomotor and postural recovery following neurologic injury. The challenge to recover these sensorimotor abilities is based on critical components: activity-dependent plasticity, the need for appropriate sensory inputs, task-specific training, repetition, and practice, and continual challenges to neuromotor adaptation to maximize recovery. Principles of locomotor and postural training have emerged from basic science findings and are translated into clinical practice, as will be described in Chapters 3 through 8.

SCI has been a model from which to understand the neural control of walking in basic science research of both animal models and the parallel human condition. This knowledge about the control of walking and activity-dependent plasticity has led to the development of rehabilitation training programs, such as Locomotor Training, to promote recovery of function. While the discussion has focused on SCI and stroke, it is conceivable that Locomotor Training is applicable to other neurologic populations with resultant walking dysfunction (Giesser et al., 2007). Good clinical judgment in combination with the scientific evidence, the client's preferences, and resources will provide the appropriate opportunity for the extension of Locomotor Training to advance recovery of walking in other types of neurologic injury and disease. In addition, autonomic function, health, and quality of life, simultaneously affected by neurologic injury and disease, may also be improved.

References

Anderson KD (2004). Targeting recovery: priorities of the spinal cord-injured population. J Neurotrauma 21: 1371–1383.

Asanuma A and Pavlides C (1997). Neurobiological basis of motor learning in mammals. NeuroReports 8: 1–6.

Barbeau H, Chau C, and Rossignol S (1993). Noradrenergic agonists and locomotor training affect locomotor recovery after cord transection in adult cats. Brain Res Bull 30: 387–393.

Barbeau H, Fung J, and Visintin M (1998a). New approach to retrain gait in stroke and spinal cord injured subjects. Neurorehab Neural Rep 13: 177–178.

Barbeau H, Nadeau S, and Garneau C (2006). Physical determinants, emerging concepts, and training approaches in gait of individuals with spinal cord injury. J Neurotrauma 23: 571–585.

Barbeau H, Norman K, Fung J, et al. (1998b). Does neurorehabilitation play a role in the recovery of walking in neurological populations? Ann N Y Acad Sci 860: 377–392.

Barbeau H, Ladouceur M, Norman K, et al. (1999). Walking after spinal cord injury: evaluation, treatment, and functional recovery. Arch Phys Med Rehabil 80: 225–235.

Barbeau H and Rossignol S (1987). Recovery of locomotion after chronic spinalization in the adult cat. Brain Res 412: 84–95.

Behrman AK, Lawless-Dixon AR, Davis SB, et al. (2005). Locomotor training progression and outcomes after incomplete spinal cord injury. Phys Ther 85: 1356–1371.

Behrman AL and Harkema SJ (2000). Locomotor training after human spinal cord injury: a series of case studies. Phys Ther 80: 688–700.

Belanger M, Drew T, Provencher J, et al. (1996). A comparison of treadmill locomotion in adult cats before and after spinal transection. J Neurophysiol 76: 471–491.

Beres-Jones JA and Harkema SJ (2004). The human spinal cord interprets velocity-dependent afferent input during stepping. Brain 127: 2232–2246.

Beres-Jones JA, Johnson TD, and Harkema SJ (2003). Clonus after human spinal cord injury cannot be attributed solely to recurrent muscle-tendon stretch. Exp Brain Res 149: 222–236.

Bouyer L and Rossignol S (1998). The contribution of cutaneous inputs to locomotion in the intact and the spinal cat. Ann N Y Acad Sci 860: 508–512.

Bouyer LJ, Whelan PJ, Pearson KG, et al. (2001). Adaptive locomotor plasticity in chronic spinal cats after ankle extensors neurectomy. J Neurosci 21: 3531–3541.

Burns SP, Golding DG, Rolle JWA, et al. (1997). Recovery of ambulation in motor-incomplete tetraplegia. Arch Phys Med Rehabil 78: 1169–1172.

Bussel B, Roby-Brami A, Neris OR, et al. (1996). Evidence for a spinal stepping generator in man. Paraplegia 34: 91–92.

Bussel B, Roby-Brami A, Yakovleff A, et al. (1989). Late flexion reflex in paraplegic patients. Evidence for a spinal stepping generator. Brain Res Bull 22: 53–56.

Calancie B, Needham-Shropshire B, Jacobs P, et al. (1994). Involuntary stepping after chronic spinal cord injury. Evidence for a central rhythm generator for locomotion in man. Brain 117(Pt 5): 1143–1159.

Carrier L, Brustein E, and Rossignol S (1997). Locomotion of the hindlimbs after neurectomy of ankle flexors in intact and spinal cats: model for the study of locomotor plasticity. J Neurophysiol 77: 1979–1993.

Chau C, Barbeau H, and Rossignol S (1998). Effects of intrathecal alpha1 and alpha2 noradrenergic agonists and norepinephrine on locomotion in chronic spinal cats. J Neurophysiol 79: 2941–2963.

Crozier KS, Cheng LL, Graziani V, et al. (1992). Spinal cord injury: prognosis for ambulation based on quadriceps recovery. Paraplegia 30: 762–767.

Curt A and Dietz V (1999). Neurologic recovery in SCI. Arch Phys Med Rehabil 80: 607–608.

Dean CM, Channon EF, and Hall JM (2007). Sitting training early after stroke improves sitting ability and quality and carries over to standing up but not to walking: a randomised trial. Aust J Physiother 53: 97–102.

de Guzman CP, Roy, RR, Hodgson, JA, et al. (1991). Coordination of motor pools controlling the ankle musculature in adult spinal cats during treadmill walking. Brain Res 555: 202–214.

de Leon RD, Hodgson JA, Roy RR, et al. (1998a). Locomotor capacity attributable to step training versus spontaneous recovery after spinalization in adult cats. J Neurophysiol 79: 1329–1340.

de Leon RD, Hodgson JA, Roy RR, et al. (1998b). Full weight-bearing hindlimb standing following stand training in the adult spinal cat. J Neurophysiol 80: 83–91.

de Leon RD, Hodgson JA, Roy RR, et al. (1999a). Retention of hindlimb stepping ability in adult spinal cats after the cessation of step training. J Neurophysiol 81: 85–94.

de Leon RD, London NJS, Roy RR, et al. (1999b). Failure analysis of stepping in adult cats. Prog Brain Res 123: 341–348.

de Leon RD, Tamaki H, Hodgson JA, et al. (1999c). Hindlimb locomotor and postural training modulates glycinergic inhibition in the spinal cord of the adult cat. J. Neurophysiol 82: 359–369.

Dietz V (1987). Role of peripheral afferents and spinal reflexes in normal and impaired human locomotion. Rev Neurol (Paris) 143: 241–254.

Dietz V (1996). Interaction between central programs and afferent input in the control of posture and locomotion. J Biomech 29: 841–844.

Dietz V (1998). Evidence for a load receptor contribution to the control of posture and locomotion. Neurosci Biobehav Rev 22: 495–499.

Dietz V (2001). Spinal cord lesion: effects of and perspectives for treatment. Neural Plast 8: 83–90.

Dietz V (2009). Body weight supported gait training: from laboratory to clinical setting. Brain Res Bull 78: I–VI.

Dietz V and Colombo G (2004). Recovery from spinal cord injury: underlying mechanisms and efficacy of rehabilitation. Acta Neurochir Suppl 89: 95–100.

Dietz V, Colombo G, and Jensen L (1994). Locomotor activity in spinal man. Lancet 344: 1260–1263.

Dietz V, Colombo G, Jensen L, et al. (1995). Locomotor capacity of spinal cord in paraplegic patients. Ann Neurol 37: 574–582.

Dietz V, Gollhofer A, Kleiber M, et al. (1992). Regulation of bipedal stance: dependency on "load" receptors. Exp Brain Res 89: 229–231.

Dietz V and Harkema, SJ (2004). Locomotor activity in spinal cord-injured persons. J Appl Physiol 96: 1954–1960.

Dietz V, Muller R, and Colombo G (2002). Locomotor activity in spinal man: significance of afferent input from joint and load receptors. Brain 125: 2626–2634.

Dietz V, Wirz M, Colombo G, et al. (1998). Locomotor capacity and recovery of spinal cord function in paraplegic patients: a clinical and electrophysiological evaluation. Electroencephalogr Clin Neurophysiol 109(2): 140–153.

Dietz V, Wirz M, and Jensen L (1997). Locomotion in patients with spinal cord injuries. Phys Ther 77: 508–516.

Dimitrijevic MR, Gerasimenko Y, and Pinter MM (1998). Evidence for a spinal central pattern generator in humans. Ann N Y Acad Sci 860: 360–376.

Ditunno J and Scivoletto G (2009). Clinical relevance of gait research applied to clinical trials in spinal cord injury. Brain Res Bull 78: 35–42.

Dobkin B, Apple D, Barbeau H, et al. (2006). Weight-supported treadmill vs. overground training for walking after acute incomplete SCI. Neurology 66: 484–493.

Dobkin BH, Harkema S, Requejo P, et al. (1995). Modulation of locomotor-like EMG activity in subjects with complete and incomplete spinal cord injury. J Neurol Rehabil 9: 183–190.

Duncan PW (2007). Barriers to evidence-based physical therapist practice for people after stroke: invited commentary. Phys Ther 83: 1304.

Duysens J, Bastiaanse CM, Smits-Engelsman BC, et al. (2004). Gait acts as a gate for reflexes from the foot. Can J Physiol Pharmacol 82: 715–722.

Duysens J, Clarac F, and Cruse H (2000). Load-regulating mechanisms in gait and posture: comparative aspects. Physiol Rev 80: 83–133.

Duysens J, Trippel M, Horstmann GA, et al. (1990). Gating and reversal of reflexes in ankle muscles during human walking. Exp Brain Res 82: 351–358.

Duysens J, van Wezel BM, van de Crommert HW, et al. (1998). The role of afferent feedback in the control of hamstrings activity during human gait. Eur J Morphol 36: 293–299.

Edgerton VR, Roy RR, Hodgson JA, et al. (1991). A physiological basis for the development of rehabilitative strategies for spinally injured patients. J Am Paraplegia Soc 14: 150–157.

Edgerton VR, Roy RR, Hodgson JA, et al. (1992). Potential of adult mammalian lumbosacral spinal cord to execute and acquire improved locomotion in the absence of supraspinal input. J Neurotrauma 9: S119–S128.

Ferris DP, Gordon KE, Beres-Jones JA, et al. (2004). Muscle activation during unilateral stepping occurs in the nonstepping limb of humans with clinically complete spinal cord injury. Spinal Cord 42: 14–23.

Finch L, Barbeau H, and Arsenault B (1991). Influence of body weight support on normal human gait: development of a gait retraining strategy. Phys Ther 71: 842–856.

Forrest GF Sisto SA, Barbeau H, et al. (2008). Neuromotor and musculoskeletal responses to locomotor training for an individual with chronic motor complete AIS-B spinal cord injury. J Spinal Cord Med 31(5): 509–521.

Forssberg H (1979a). On integrative motor functions in the cat's spinal cord. Acta Physiol Scand 474: 1–56.

Forssberg H (1979b). Stumbling corrective reaction: a phase-dependent compensatory reaction during locomotion. J Neurophysiol 42(4): 936–953.

Forssberg H, Grillner S, Halbertsma J, et al. (1980). The locomotion of the low spinal cat. II. interlimb coordination. Acta Physiol Scand 108: 283–295.

Forssberg H, Grillner S, and Rossignol S (1977). Phasic gain control of reflexes from the dorsum of the paw during spinal locomotion. Brain Res 132: 121–139.

Fouad K and Pearson K (2004). Restoring walking after spinal cord injury. Prog Neurobiol 73(2): 107–126.

Gerasimenko YP, Makarovskii AN, and Nikitin OA (2002). Control of locomotor activity in humans and animals in the absence of supraspinal influences. Neurosci Behav Physiol 32(4): 417–423.

Giesser B, Beres-Jones J, Budovitch A, et al. (2007). Locomotor training using body weight support on a treadmill improves mobility in persons with multiple sclerosis: pilot study. Mult Scler 13: 224–231.

Gorassini MA, Norton JA, Nevett-Duchcherer J, et al. (2009). Changes in locomotor muscle activity after training in subjects with incomplete spinal cord injury. J. Neurophysiol 101(2): 969–979.

Grasso R, Ivanenko YP, Zago M, et al. (2004). Recovery of forward stepping in spinal-cord injured patients does not transfer to untrained backward stepping. Exp Brain Res 157(3): 377–382.

Grillner S (1981). Control of locomotion in bipeds, tetrapods, and fish. In: Handbook of Physiology: The Nervous System II. Bethesda, MD: American Physiological Society, 1179–1236.

Grillner S and Rossignol S (1978). On the initiation of the swing phase of locomotion in chronic spinal cats. Brain Res 146: 269–277.

Hannold EM, Young ME, Rittman MR, et al. (2006). Locomotor training: experiencing the changing body. J Rehabil Res Dev 43(7): 905–916.

Harkema SJ (2001). Neural plasticity after human spinal cord injury: application of locomotor training to the rehabilitation of walking. Neuroscientists 7(5): 455–468.

Harkema SJ (2008). Plasticity of interneuronal networks of the functionally isolated human spinal cord. Brain Res Rev 57: 255–264.

Harkema SJ, Ferreira CK, van den Brand RJ, et al. (2008). Improvements in orthostatic instability with stand locomotor training in individuals with spinal cord injury. J Neurotrauma 25(12): 1467–1475.

Harkema SJ, Hurley SL, Patel UK, et al. (1997). Human lumbosacral spinal cord interprets loading during stepping. J Neurophysiol 77: 797–811.

Harkema SJ, Schmidt-Read, Lorenz DL, et al (2011). Establishing the NeuroRecovery Network: Balance and ambulation improvements in individuals with chronic incomplete spinal cord injury using Locomotor Training- based rehabilitation. Arch Phys Med Rehabil *In Press*.

Hesse S, Helm MD, Krajnik J, et al. (1997). Treadmill training with partial body weight support: influence of body weight release on the gait of hemiparetic patients. J Neurol Rehab 11(1): 15–20.

Hesse S, Helm MD, Krajnik J, et al. (1999). Treadmill training with partial body weight support versus floor walking in hemiparetic patients. Arch Phys Med Rehabil 80(4): 421–427.

Hesse S, Bertfelt C, Jahnke MT et al. (1995). Treadmill training with partial body weight support compared with physiotherapy in nonambulatory hemiparetic patients. Stroke 26(6): 976–981.

Hesse S, Bertfelt C, Schaffrin A et al. (1994). Restoration of gait in nonambulatory hemiparetic patients by treadmill training with partial body-weight support. Arch Phys Med Rehabil 75: 1087–1093.

Hicks AL, Adams MM, Martin Ginis K, et al. (2005). Long-term body-weight-supported treadmill training and subsequent follow-up in persons with chronic SCI: effects on functional walking ability and measures of subjective well being. Spinal Cord 43(5): 291–298.

Hornby TG, Campbell DD, Hahn JH, et al. (2008). Enhanced gait-related improvements after therapists- versus robotic-assisted locomotor training in subjects with chronic stroke: a randomized controlled study. Stroke 39(6): 1786–1792.

Hussey RW and Stauffer ES (1973). Spinal cord injury: requirements for ambulation. Arch Phys Med Rehabil 54: 544–547.

Jankowska E (1992). Interneuronal relay in spinal pathways from proprioceptors. Prog Neurobiol 38: 335–378.

Jankowska E and Riddell JS (1995). Interneurones mediating presynaptic inhibition of group II muscle afferents in the cat spinal cord. J Physiol 483(Pt 2): 461–471.

Jayaraman A, Shah P, Gregory C, et al. (2008). Locomotor training and muscle function after incomplete spinal cord injury: cases series. J Spinal Cord Med 31(2): 185–193.

Johansson BB, Haker E, von AM, et al. (2001). Acupuncture and transcutaneous nerve stimulation in stroke rehabilitation: a randomized, controlled trial. Stroke 32: 707–713.

Kojima N, Nakazawa K, and Yano H (1999). Effects of limb loading on the lower-limb electromyographic activity during orthotic locomotion in a paraplegic patient. Neurosci Lett 274: 211–213.

Kosak MC and Reding MJ (2000). Comparison of partial body weight-supported treadmill gait training versus aggressive bracing assisted walking post stroke. Neurorehabil Neural Repair 14: 13–19.

Kuhn RA (1950). Functional capacity of the isolated human spinal cord. Brain 73(1): 1–51.

Ladouceur M and Barbeau H (2000a). Functional electrical stimulation-assisted walking for persons with incomplete spinal injuries: longitudinal changes in maximal overground walking speed. Scand J Rehabil Med 32: 28–36.

Ladouceur M and Barbeau H (2000b). Functional electrical stimulation-assisted walking for persons with incomplete spinal injuries: changes in the kinematics and physiological cost of overground walking. Scand J Rehabil Med 32: 72–79.

Lewek MD, Cruz TH, Moore JL, et al. (2009). Allowing intralimb kinematic variability during locomotor training poststroke improves kinematic consistency: a subgroup analysis from a randomized clinical trial. Phys Ther 89(8): 829–839.

Lovely R, Gregor R, Roy RR, et al. (1986). Effects of training on the recovery of full-weight bearing stepping in the adult spinal cat. Exp Neurol 92: 421–435.

Lovely R, Gregor R, Roy RR, et al. (1990). Weight bearing hindlimb stepping in treadmill-exercised adult spinal cats. Brain Res 514: 206–218.

Lunenburger L, Bolliger M, Czell D, et al. (2006). Modulation of locomotor activity in complete spinal cord injury. Exp Brain Res 174: 638–646.

Maegele M, Muller S, Wernig A, et al. (2002). Recruitment of spinal motor pools during voluntary movements versus stepping after human spinal cord injury. J Neurotrauma 19: 1217–1229.

Marino RJ, Barros T, Biering-Sorensen F, et al. (2003). International standards for neurological classification of spinal cord injury. J Spinal Cord Med 26(1): S50–S56.

McCrea DA (2001). Spinal circuitry of sensorimotor control of locomotion. J Physiol 533: 41–50.

Moseley AM, Stark A, Cameron ID, et al. (2005). Treadmill training and body weight support for walking after stroke. Cochrane Database Syst Rev CD002840.

Mulroy S, Gronley J, Weiss W, et al. (2003). Use of cluster analysis for gait pattern classification of patients in the early and late recovery phases following stroke. Gait Posture 18: 114–125.

Nadeau S, Arsenault AB, Gravel D, et al. (1999). Analysis of the clinical factors determining natural and maximal gait speeds in adults with a stroke. Am J Phys Med Rehabil 78: 123–130.

Nilsson L, Carlsson J, Danielsson A, et al. (2001). Walking training of patients with hemiparesis at an early stage after stroke: a comparison of walking training on a treadmill with body weight support and walking training on the ground. Clin Rehabil 15: 515–527.

Pearson KG (2004). Generating the walking gait: role of sensory feedback. Prog Brain Res 143: 123–129.

Phillips SM, Stewart BG, Mahoney DJ, et al. (2004). Body-weight-support treadmill training improves blood glucose regulation in persons with incomplete spinal cord injury. J Appl Physiol 97(2): 716–724.

Pohl M, Mehrholz J, Ritschel C, et al. (2002). Speed-dependent treadmill training in ambulatory hemiparetic stroke patients: a randomized controlled trial. Stroke 33: 553–558.

Roopchand S, Fung J, and Barbeau H (2005) Locomotor training and the effects of unloading on overground locomotion following stroke. In: Brown SP (Ed.), Focus on Stroke Research. Nova Science Publishers, 169–189.

Rossignol S (2000). Locomotion and its recovery after spinal injury. Curr Opin Neurobiol 10: 708–716.

Rossignol S, Barbeau H, and Julien C (1986). Locomotion of the adult chronic spinal cat and its modification by monoaminergic agonists and antagonists. In: Golberger ME, Gario A, and Murray M (Eds.), Development and Plasticity of the Mammalian Spinal Cord. Fidia Research Series, vol. 111. Liviana Press Padova Springer Verlag, 323–345.

Rossignol S, Bouyer L, Barthelemy D, et al. (2002). Recovery of locomotion in the cat following spinal cord lesions. Brain Res Brain Res Rev 40(1–3): 257–266.

Rossignol S, Chau C, Brustein E, et al (1996). Locomotor capacities after complete and partial lesions of the spinal cord. Acta Neurobiol Exp 56: 449–463.

Rossignol S, Dubuc R, and Gossard JP (2006). Dynamic sensorimotor interactions in locomotion. Physiol Rev 86: 89–154.

Shepherd RE and Carr J (1999). Treadmill walking in neurorehabilitation. Neurorehabil Neural Repair 13: 171–173.

Sherrington SCS (1900). On the innervation of antagonistic muscles. Sixth note. Proc Royal Soc 66: 66–75.

Sherwood AM, Dimitrijevic MR, and McKay WB (1992). Evidence of subclinical brain influence in clinically complete spinal cord injury: discomplete SCI. J Neurol Sci 110: 90–98.

Sinkjaer T, Andersen JB, and Larsen B (1996). Soleus stretch reflex modulation during gait in humans. J Neurophysiol 76: 1112–1120.

Sullivan KJ, Knowlton BJ, and Dobkin BH (2002). Step training with body weight support: effect of treadmill speed and practice paradigms on poststroke locomotor recovery. Arch Phys Med Rehabil 83: 683–691.

Tremblay F, Malouin F, Richards CL, et al. (1990). Effects of prolonged muscle stretch on reflex and voluntary muscle activations in children with spastic cerebral palsy. Scand J Rehabil Med 22: 171–180.

Vilensky JA and O'Connor BL (1997). Stepping in humans with complete spinal cord transection: a phylogenetic evaluation. Motor Control 1: 284–292.

Visintin M and Barbeau H (1989). The effects of body weight support on the locomotor pattern of spastic paretic patients. Can J Neurol Sci 16: 315–325.

Visintin M, Barbeau H, Korner-Bitensky N, et al. (1998). A new approach to retrain gait in stroke patients through body weight support and treadmill stimulation. Stroke 29: 1122–1128.

Waters RL, Adkins RH, Yakura JS, et al. (1994). Motor and sensory recovery following incomplete paraplegia. Arch Phys Med Rehabil 75: 67–72.

Waters RL, Yakura JS, and Adkins RH (1993). Gait performance after spinal cord injury. Clin Orthop Relat Res 288: 87–96.

Wernig A and Müller S (1992). Laufband locomotion with body weight support improved walking in persons with severe spinal cord injuries. Paraplegia 30: 229–238.

Wernig A, Müller S, Nanassy A, et al. (1995). Laufband therapy based on "rules of spinal locomotion" is effective in spinal cord injured persons. Eur J Neurosci 7: 823–829.

Winstein CJ, Gardner ER, McNeal DR, et al. (1989). Standing balance training: effect on balance and locomotion in hemiparetic adults. Arch Phys Med Rehabil 70: 755–762.

Wirz M, Colombo G, and Dietz V (2001). Long-term effects of locomotor training in spinal humans. J Neurol Neurosurg Physch 71(1): 93–96.

Yang JF, Fung J, Edamura M, et al. (1991). H-reflex modulation during walking in spastic paretic subjects. Can J Neurol Sci 18: 443–452.

Yang JF, Lamont EV, and Pang MY (2005). Split-belt treadmill stepping in infants suggests autonomous pattern generators for the left and right leg in humans. J Neurosci 25: 6869–6876.

Yang JF, Stephens MJ, and Vishram R (1998). Infant stepping: a method to study the sensory control of human walking. J Physiol 507(Pt 3): 927–937.

Zehr EP, Komiyama T, and Stein RB (1997). Cutaneous reflexes during human gait: electromyographic and kinematic responses to electrical stimulation. J Neurophysiol 77: 3311–3325.

3

Locomotor Training as an Activity-Based Therapy for Posture, Standing, and Walking

Chapter Outline

Chapter Objectives

The objectives of Chapter 3 are to:

1. Define functional goals and recovery of function and understand their differences.
2. Define *activity-based therapy*.
3. Define *Locomotor Training*.
4. Recall the four Locomotor Training principles and provide examples.
5. State the three components of Locomotor Training and the goal of each.
6. List the four phases of recovery for locomotion.
7. List the four areas of progression in retraining the neural capacity and adapting to functional tasks.
8. Describe the clinical model for delivery of Locomotor Training.

Summary

This chapter will present the concepts that have facilitated the translation of scientific evidence for activity-dependent plasticity into the clinical implementation of an activity-based therapy, Locomotor Training. We will discuss the paradigm shift from compensation-based rehabilitation to activity-based therapy. We will present the four guiding principles that serve as the basis for clinical decisions throughout the three components of Locomotor Training to facilitate clients to continually recover function while achieving functional goals at home and advancing through the phases of recovery.

Compensation-Based Rehabilitation to Activity-Based Therapy

Spinal cord injury (SCI) and stroke reduce the ability of individuals to walk in their homes and communities. This consequently reduces their physical activity and has a negative impact on their health (see Chapter 1). Diminished access to the community decreases their ability to fully participate in society and reduces their quality of life. While the etiology of gait dysfunction differs between the two groups, there are commonalities in the response of the neuromuscular system to solving the problem of locomotion. If walking is possible, usually overall walking speed is slower and the ability to adapt to the demands of the environment is severely compromised. To be able to walk again after experiencing SCI, stroke, or other neurologic insult is a primary goal for many individuals.

Compensation Approaches

The focus of rehabilitation has been on accomplishing a functional task by compensating for impairments. Behavioral compensation refers to the recruitment of additional body segments or systems, or an integration of alternative motor elements, or equipment (e.g., wheelchair, assistive device, gait orthoses) to compensate for neuromuscular deficits to achieve a daily task and functional goal. This may include the overuse of one segment or system for the underuse of another or may result in a functional goal achieved by different end effectors or body segments. For example, greater movements at the trunk, hip, or pelvis can compensate for inability to advance the legs. The use of braces and assistive devices has been introduced to further compensate for sensorimotor impairments after incomplete SCI and stroke to achieve the goal of mobility. While the immediate functional goal of ambulation may be achieved with compensation, the therapeutic effect on recovery of neuromuscular function may be delayed because addressing the neural source of the deficit is a secondary focus.

For instance, Michael, an individual with an incomplete SCI, walked using a walker. When asked to attempt to walk without the walker he responded, "But I was taught to walk again with six legs, not two"—his own two legs and the four legs of the walker. That comment embodies the strategies that have guided rehabilitation and enablement of achieving functional goals for ambulation after SCI. The walker, in this example, was a means to the end. Rehabilitation did not restore the premorbid function of this individual's neuromuscular system to achieve walking but did enable the individual to advance overground. The walker distributed load-bearing between the arms and the legs to achieve balance and afford upright mobility. This strategy compensated for weak legs, uncoordinated leg movement, and insufficient control of the trunk and posture during standing and walking and reduced the risk of falling. The *functional goal*, ambulation, was accomplished; however, how the task was performed represents a novel movement pattern, not *recovery of function* for locomotion.

Recovery refers to restoration of the neuromuscular system to regain function of a specific motor task and the reacquisition of elemental motor behaviors as performed before the injury. While compensation has been the mainstay of rehabilitation for years, the potential for restoration of neuromuscular function (below the level of the lesion after SCI) via premorbid movement patterns recently has been demonstrated in laboratories and clinics (see Chapter 2). New knowledge of the neurobiologic control of walking and the plasticity of the nervous system in response to repetitive and challenging activity is reshaping the direction of physical rehabilitation after neurologic injury. Partnerships of basic scientists, clinicians, and applied scientists, as exemplified in this text, have resulted in translation of such knowledge from the laboratory to the human condition and have formed the basis for activity-based therapies. Physical rehabilitation is embarking on a new era with a paradigm shift in our thinking and clinical decision making from a primary focus on compensation to now emphasizing activity-based therapy.

Activity-Based Therapy

In the scientific literature, *activity-dependent plasticity* is a term that indicates changes in the nervous or muscular systems that are driven by repetitive activity (refer to Chapter 2). In the context of Locomotor Training, retraining is based on activity-dependent plasticity driven by repetitive task-specific sensory input to spinal networks and the neural axis. Studies show that the spinal cord integrates supraspinal and afferent information and with repetitive practice can improve motor output. With the translation of these scientific findings to the human condition, rehabilitation strategies emerged that use the intrinsic properties of the nervous system in response to task-specific activity to advance and improve recovery of function after SCI.

Activity-based therapy specifically refers to interventions that focus on recovery by providing activation of the neuromuscular system below the level of the lesion with the goal of retraining the individual to recover function of a specific motor task. Locomotor Training is an activity-based therapy that promotes recovery of walking and other motor functions by taking advantage of intrinsic neural mechanisms of the nervous system to promote an effective locomotor output. The primary goal of Locomotor Training is to provide appropriate sensory cues to retrain neural activation patterns that will result in effective posture, standing, and walking. With diminished supraspinal input, the nervous system must rely more heavily on the interneuronal networks and the clarity of sensory information that is specific to the task of walking in order to recover this function. A series of guiding principles for training has emerged in the translation of findings from basic science to the human condition.

In the previous example, for Michael to recover walking using two legs and not "six," three fundamental, sensorimotor control tasks would need to be restored: (1) a reciprocal stepping pattern (e.g., limb load, support, transition from stance to swing, swing, and transition to loading), (2) dynamic balance and postural control during walking, and (3) adaptation of the walking pattern and postural control to meet the demands of the environment (e.g., inclines, curbs, uneven terrain) and his own behavioral goals (e.g., carrying a backpack, hurrying to cross a busy street). Locomotor Training was developed to accomplish these tasks by applying specific therapeutic components targeting progression areas that guide individuals such as Michael through the four phases of recovery.

Locomotor Training Principles

The four fundamental guiding principles of Locomotor Training are built on the premise of robustly providing appropriate sensory cues to the spinal networks that are involved in walking through repetitive practice and integrating the new capacity and recovery to reach functional goals. Following these principles will optimize sensory input related to walking, thereby optimizing the development of neural patterns for locomotion and minimizing compensation strategies. The principles are emphasized throughout the book and should be used in the clinical setting whenever decisions are made by the clinicians during treatment and by the client in the home and community. Here the four Locomotor Training principles are briefly introduced with some examples of application.

Throughout the remaining chapters, application of these principles to promote recovery and examples will be addressed in detail.

Maximize Weight-Bearing on the Legs (Principle 1)

In all components of Locomotor Training, weight-bearing plays a critical role in retraining the nervous system and in progressing the individual to the next phase of recovery. The therapists and trainers should continuously identify strategies to bear as much body weight as possible with the legs. During the therapeutic intervention, trainers should identify opportunities to maximize the total time the individual is weight-bearing, such as standing while applying the harness and when discussing goals or explaining the details of a particular session. During the step training component, the trainer should lower the body weight support (BWS) whenever feasible throughout the stepping and standing bouts. When transferring, the trainer should always place the client's feet on the floor and emphasize weight-bearing on the legs while minimizing weight-bearing on the arms. Finally, the trainer should encourage standing in the home and community (e.g., stand as often as possible, such as while brushing teeth, washing dishes, or pushing a grocery cart). Loading of the legs is a powerful sensory cue that when intensely used can lead to the progression of recovery of standing and walking; it should be considered during acute care and throughout the continuum of recovery.

Optimize Sensory Cues Appropriate for Specific Motor Task (Principle 2)

The success of task-specific training relies on the appropriate sensory cues being sent back to the spinal cord related to posture, standing, and walking. This includes weight-bearing and kinematics as well as the rate at which the information is delivered. The intrinsic spinal circuitry is more reliant on these cues when supraspinal input is compromised and thus the afferent input has more influence on the final motor output. This can be observed, for example, when spasticity is sometimes set off simply by pinching the skin. Thus, when retraining walking, it is important to spend considerable time stepping at estimated pre-injury walking speeds to provide the expected sensory information. Critical sensory cues related to hip extension and unloading of the leg can be used to initiate swing when voluntary control is too impaired. Also, stimulating flexor and extensor tendons at the appropriate time in the step cycle can activate these muscles during stance and swing, respectively, to facilitate the retraining of the nervous system.

Optimize Kinematics for Each Motor Task (Principle 3)

Facilitating the proper kinematics for standing, stepping, and other motor tasks generates the appropriate sensory information essential for driving neural recovery. Focus should be on maintaining upright posture of the head, trunk, and position of the pelvis during standing and walking. During walking effective extension and flexion of the hip, knee, and ankle and facilitation of interlimb and intralimb coordination is needed during retraining of stepping. This focus is especially important to avoid reinforcing compensatory strategies that use abnormal kinematics to accomplish similar mobility goals. In addition, when completing any motor task, maintaining the correct kinematics and kinetics will capitalize on the intrinsic capacity of the nervous system to execute the movement.

Maximize Recovery Strategies; Minimize Compensation Strategies (Principle 4)

Activity-dependent plasticity occurs continuously and the nervous system will change based on the information received and the tasks practiced. Compensation strategies can lead to the nervous system changing in response to assistance provided, either resulting in routine motor patterns such as hip hiking and circumduction or limiting recovery of activation of a specific joint. Thus, Locomotor Training strongly emphasizes maximizing recovery and minimizing compensation by always promoting independence before providing assistance in every motor task. Therapists and trainers should instruct and encourage the client to attempt motor tasks independently before assisting. A movement strategy should be used that closely approximates the specific motor task while minimizing use of compensation strategies. The least restrictive assistive devices should be selected that are most consistent with the Locomotor Training principles, and they should be used only when needed for independence, endurance, and safety.

Locomotor Training Therapeutic Components

There are three key components to Locomotor Training: step training (Fig. 3-1a), overground assessment (Fig. 3.1b), and community integration (Fig. 3.1c). The ultimate goal of Locomotor Training is for clients to achieve independent mobility and walking in the

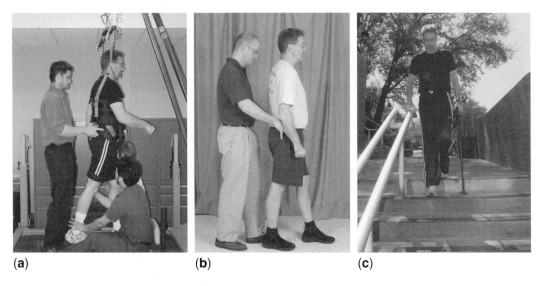

(a)   **(b)**   **(c)**

FIG 3-1 Locomotor training components. **a.** Step training on the treadmill (from Sisto et al., 2009, with permission from Elsevier). **b.** Assessment overground (from Sisto et al., 2009, with permission from Elsevier). **c.** Community integration.

home and community and to improve their health and quality of life after neurologic injury by inducing recovery of function. Walking is a complex task composed of stepping movements, balance (postural control/dynamic stability), and response to environmental demands. Retraining the nervous system to achieve targeted motor tasks primarily occurs during *step training* using body weight support on the treadmill (BWST) and manual facilitation. Recovery of function here is then translated to mobility and walking in the home and community. Limitations and gait deviations identified during *overground assessment* are set as primary goals for retraining. These goals are also addressed with targeted activities for home and community and are identified and practiced during *community integration*. These goals are then addressed in the next step training session. Thus, the three components of Locomotor Training are integrated for the client to achieve maximum recovery. All three components are addressed in each therapy session beginning with step training and followed by overground walking assessment and community integration. Goals in each component are modified continuously, based on the phase of recovery and progress made within and across Locomotor Training components.

Step Training

The goal of step training is to retrain individuals to stand and generate stepping movements by taking advantage of the intrinsic mechanisms of the nervous system that generate neuromuscular activity. The nervous system eventually reorganizes to generate effective motor patterns associated with standing and walking. Step training uses a BWST system in combination with manual facilitation by trainers to implement the Locomotor Training principles. An overhead safety cable with the BWS system ensures client confidence and safety and prevents falling. The treadmill speed, partial BWS, and manual facilitation by trainers can be controlled to optimally provide sensory cues repetitively for extensive practice (retraining) and challenge to the nervous system to be independent (adaptability). Step training using BWST and manual facilitation is also used to address limitations to independent walking, including gait deviations, and to promote independence and balance.

Four distinct approaches are used during the step training session: (1) stand retraining, (2) step retraining, (3) stand adaptability, and (4) step adaptability. The stand and step retraining bouts of the session focus on repetitively providing the optimal sensory cues for the specific task. The primary focus for stand retraining is to continually increase weight-bearing while maintaining the proper posture and positioning for standing using manual facilitation at the trunk, pelvis, and legs as needed. Stepping at normal walking speeds is prioritized during step retraining, and then the goal is to reduce the amount of BWS while maintaining the appropriate kinematics for stepping using manual facilitation. The primary focus for the stand adaptability and step adaptability bouts is to promote independence during standing and stepping by varying the BWS level and treadmill speed. The majority of the step training component is devoted to retraining, with the time spent in step retraining always exceeding the time spent in stand retraining. The focus of step and stand adaptability varies based on the phase of recovery (see Chapter 7) and the progression goals (see Chapter 8).

Overground Assessment

The goal of overground assessment is to understand the neuromuscular capacity for mobility, standing, and walking without the BWST and manual facilitation (see Chapter 7 for details). Specific tasks are evaluated, such as sitting upright, moving from supine to a sitting position, laying down from the sitting position to supine, transitioning from sitting to standing, standing, and walking. Limitations to independent mobility, posture, standing, and walking are identified and specifically targeted in the next step training session, where the BWST environment allows easier intervention by the trainer. These limitations may also be addressed in home- and community-based activities to further advance recovery.

Community Integration

The goal of community integration is to translate the stepping and neuromuscular capacity gained by retraining the nervous system during step training into safe overground mobility, standing and walking in the home and community, and performing everyday activities. The Locomotor Training principles used during step training are also used to promote daily function, standing, and walking outside of the clinical environment. If required, the therapist selects the least restrictive assistive device that provides safe and independent ambulation. The client is instructed on strategies to use the device in a manner that is consistent with the principles. The client is also instructed on strategies to safely function in the home environment without the assistive device and during other everyday activities.

Phases of Recovery

The Phases of Recovery are used by the physical therapist to evaluate the client's neural capacity for mobility, standing, and walking (see Chapter 7). The approach is to evaluate the current capacity of the nervous and musculoskeletal systems to achieve specific motor tasks. This evaluation is optimally conducted in the step training component using the BWST environment, where balance deficits are limited and fear of falling is minimized. The BWST is a permissive environment in that sensory cues are easily and effectively provided to promote activation of the neuromuscular system below the level of the lesion. In this environment, the client's response to the sensory cues for standing, stepping, and postural control are assessed. Patterns of leg muscle activation for stepping are identified during the assessment of neural capacity during the stance and swing phases of the gait cycle, as well as transitions. Based upon the findings of the evaluation, the therapist will establish goals for treatment and implement a standardized plan of care.

An additional assessment of the neural capacity for accomplishing the tasks needed for mobility, standing, and walking occurs during the assessment overground. In contrast to the BWST environment, overground the client's neural capacity is challenged in a less permissive but real-world environment. The ability of the client to perform motor tasks is assessed without the use of compensation (braces) or assistive devices while safety is maintained by manual facilitation or guarding by trainers. In addition to walking, the neural capacity to perform other functional tasks is assessed. Tasks assessed include the capacity to sit upright, sit up from supine, extend the trunk, balance during sitting, transition from sit to stand, and stand.

There are four general Phases of Recovery, defined by client ability. The phases are used to classify sensorimotor function, establish goals, progress the client and evaluate task-specific recovery.

Phase 1

Phase 1 is the earliest stage of recovery. The individual typically uses a wheelchair for mobility, is severely limited in the overground environment, and needs maximal assistance for upright mobility and ambulation (Fig. 3-2a). Often the individual experiences symptoms of multiple secondary conditions related to neurologic injury. The primary focus is retraining the nervous system to maintain an upright trunk during standing. Trunk stability and upright posture are necessary to promote leg activation and are critical for eventual walking overground.

Phase 2

Phase 2 is the mid-stage of recovery. This individual can stand but is typically non-ambulatory without bracing or assistive devices (Fig. 3-2b). The primary focus is retraining of the nervous system to stand and step and have independence in standing and begin walking. By the end of phase 2, the client should be able to stand and step with upright posture using minimal BWS.

Phase 3

Phase 3 is the late stage of recovery. The individual ambulates in the community without bracing, with or without assistive devices (Fig. 3-2c). Training focuses on increasing stepping and functional independence while decreasing dependence on assistive devices. By the end of phase 3, the client is a full-time ambulator in the community and is independent of braces and physical assistance and other compensations.

Phase 4

Phase 4 is the final stage of recovery. Having achieved independence in community ambulation, this client may be unable to adapt to the requirements for independent community mobility posed by the environment and his or her own behavioral goals (Fig. 3-2d). Safely negotiating obstacles in the overground environment (e.g., steps, uneven terrain, inclines) and the need to alter speed or stop rapidly, perform dual tasks such as walking and carrying items, and sustain walking activity for prolonged periods all pose additional neural control requirements and are the primary focus of phase 4. In addition, the client may target the goal of returning to pre-injury recreational activities that also challenge locomotor adaptability (e.g., playing basketball, running, dancing).

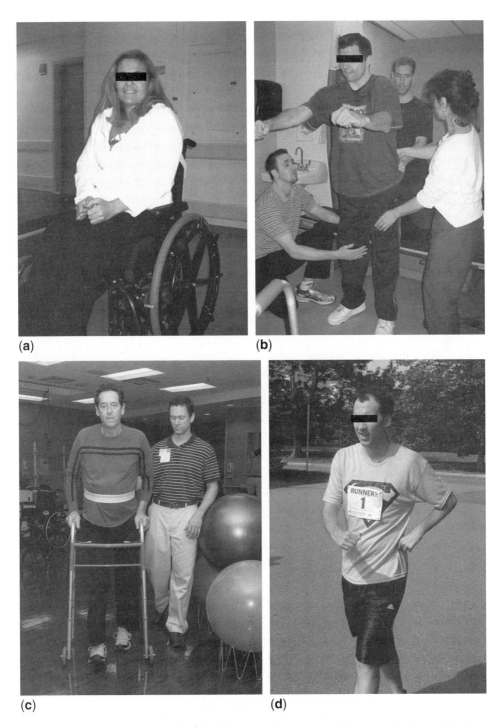

FIG 3-2 a–d. Phases of recovery. **a.** Phase 1 is the earliest stage of recovery. **b.** Phase 2 is the mid-stage of recovery. **c.** Phase 3 is the late stage of recovery. **d.** Phase 4 is the final stage of recovery.

Properly and continuously challenging clients to achieve higher levels of performance is critical to regaining locomotion. To optimize recovery and assist the client on the road to recovery, trainers must know the four areas in which progression occurs and where these areas are emphasized within the different phases of recovery. There are four general areas in which progression should occur: endurance, speed, weight-bearing (load), and independence. In addition, progression across the phases requires continuous adaptations to the increasing demands of the task of walking in varied environments. These tasks may include increasing speed, step height, and step length during steady-state walking; initiating walking and terminating walking (at various speeds); turning; climbing stairs/curbs; negotiating inclines; stepping in different directions; and carrying items while walking.

Endurance

Endurance is the ability to persist in physical activity and to resist fatigue. Within Locomotor Training, endurance is measured by (1) the total duration in minutes of activity such as standing and stepping; (2) continuous duration of stepping in minutes; and (3) the length of time an individual can independently execute a task (e.g., sitting, standing, or walking). For example, the client exhibits a greater endurance with four 5-minute bouts of stepping versus ten 2-minute bouts of stepping. Achieving the intensity of training is also critical for retraining the nervous system. Intensity is often measured by the actual amount of activity. An early goal of training is achieving adequate intensity of training (e.g., 30 minutes of stepping). As recovery progresses, endurance relates to the sustainability of an independent movement for mobility and eventually standing and walking.

Speed

Pre-injury, near-normal walking speed is more easily attained during step retraining sessions where the speed of the treadmill is set by the trainers and manual facilitation may be provided. To achieve independent stepping on the treadmill and focus on adaptability following step retraining, the treadmill speed may be slowed to the individual's capacity and increased as recovery occurs. Normal walking speed is more challenging to achieve during overground walking and community integration but is an ongoing goal for progression.

Weight-Bearing (Load)

Maximizing weight-bearing is an important principle of Locomotor Training. Weight-bearing through the legs should be progressively increased in every component. Generally, this involves increasing the load on the legs and minimizing the load on the arms during standing and stepping while in retraining, overground, and community environments.

Independence

Independence is the ultimate goal desired for the client. Independence can be defined in many ways within Locomotor Training—for example, independence from (1) manual facilitation by trainers at the hips and/or legs during step training, (2) BWS during step training, (3) wearing braces in the community, (4) assistive devices during community walking, and (5) the physical therapist or trainers during any and all phases of recovery.

Clinical Model

Equipment

The equipment used in the Locomotor Training program includes a closed-loop computer-controlled BWST system that controls treadmill speeds from 0.5 to 10 mph, seating systems that include ergonomically appropriate back and leg support designed for staff safety (Fig. 3-3), client harnesses of various sizes, front and side mirrors that provide visual feedback, a variety of assistive devices, and automatic blood pressure and heart rate monitor.

Staffing

Staffing requirements vary across the three environments (BWST, overground, and community) and as a client progresses. A ratio of one skilled therapist to three skilled technicians is an optimal staffing model for the early sessions of Locomotor Training (Fig. 3-3). Other models, such as two therapists and two activity-based therapy technicians, are acceptable but may be less cost-effective. As the client progresses, a decrease in direct

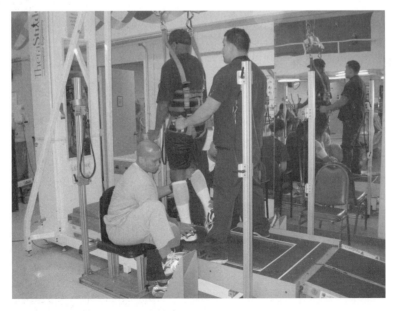

FIG 3-3 Clinical model: body weight support and treadmill equipment with ergonomic seating and staffing options.

manual facilitation is expected, potentially reducing the number of staff required for the session. This parallels other common therapeutic approaches to gait training where more than one staff member can assist with ambulation and assistive device use, although not throughout an entire therapy session. Preparation for and closure of the session and the overground assessment and community integration components require fewer staff members.

Staff may be trained with competencies specific to Locomotor Training to facilitate efficient and effective service delivery. When training clinical staff, it is important to establish clinical competency in various aspects of the training. For instance, a staff member may become competent at fitting the harness and placing the harness on a client before becoming competent as a "leg trainer." Using this book as a resource, a clinical competency checklist may be developed for each role and task as a guide during staff training and assessment of skills. Hands-on training courses paralleling this text are also available in the United States, providing a comprehensive introduction to Locomotor Training, as well as advanced skills and clinical decision making. Video feedback of training sessions is also useful to promote skill development of trainers and clinical problem solving for challenging clients. Therapists and trainers continue to advance their skills and clinical decision making with ongoing clinical experience. Working as a team to provide effective Locomotor Training requires communication and coordination among every team member.

Clinical Guidelines

Although training protocols used by researchers and clinicians vary, these guidelines represent a structured translation from basic science evidence for the neural control of walking to therapeutic principles for retraining locomotion. These guidelines will continue to be refined and clarified as research advances the science underlying Locomotor Training.

Guidelines provide a framework for clinical decision making, as well as a reference point for evaluating the potential application of any new modality, equipment, or therapeutic component. Clinical choices can be made that are consistent with the principles (i.e., no weight-bearing on the upper extremities during step training by use of overhead partial BWS) for facilitating recovery via a therapeutic effect. Thus, minimizing weight-bearing on the arms promotes loading of the legs and activation of leg muscles for support. Achievement of a therapeutic effect means that with retraining, function is restored (i.e., the legs are activated to provide weight support for upright posture and walking). Clinical choices that are inconsistent with the framework (i.e., use of a long leg brace) may reflect a choice of compensation for neuromuscular deficits and an immediate outcome of achieved mobility without a therapeutic effect. With removal of the long leg brace, there is likely no improvement in the capacity to activate limb extension.

Mastering these principles and integrating them among three components of Locomotor Training (step training on the treadmill, overground assessment, and community integration) will optimize the success realized by both the client and therapist. Progression is critical to advancing skill development and the neuromuscular capacity for walking. Training parameters are adjusted daily by adjusting the duration of stepping time, amount of BWS, speed of walking, and degree of independence in postural control and the kinematics of stepping to train and challenge the nervous system. On the road to recovery, the client progresses through four phases of recovery, each with targeted progression goals. The actual time needed for each phase of recovery will vary with each individual because the recovery process is nonlinear. Within each phase of recovery, different components of Locomotor Training are emphasized and various areas of progression are stressed.

4

Basic Skills for Implementation
of Locomotor Training

Chapter Outline

Chapter Objectives

The objectives of Chapter 4 are to:

1. Identify proper client attire and harness application.
2. State proper placement of support apparatus, including pelvic belt, harness vest, and leg straps.
3. Understand the key elements needed for a body weight support system for client and trainer safety and optimal retraining.
4. Identify the proper position of the client and the trainer at the hips and legs during standing and stepping.
5. State the important factors to consider during the four phases of stepping.
6. Describe proper coordination among trainers during the four phases of stepping.
7. State the appropriate stride length and cadence.
8. State the rationale for modified and reverse hand placements.

Summary

Successfully providing the Locomotor Training intervention is dependent on knowledge, skill, and clinical decisions for progression. Proper harness application and appropriate client attire are critical to optimizing the step training session. It is essential for therapists and trainers to understand the neurophysiologic rationale behind their positioning and hand placements so they can optimize retraining of clients' nervous systems. The attributes of the harness and body weight support on the treadmill (BWST) system are also very important for client safety, therapist and trainer protection from injury, and optimal retraining of stepping for the client.

Proper Attire, Harness Application, and Support Apparatus

Proper Client Attire

Before the client arrives for the first session, she or he should be informed of the proper attire for the therapy sessions and should be told that a support apparatus will be worn during training. Shorts are worn to expose the legs to facilitate proper hand placements by the trainers. Gym shorts or soft material that will not generate friction between the skin and harness is best (thus, not blue jeans). Male clients are encouraged to wear athletic supporters to protect the genitals from pinching and possible injury from the harness. Loose shirts are used to allow for ventilation and flexibility when placing the harness. For individuals with compromised ability to regulate temperature, layers of clothing are helpful, as they may be either abnormally cold or hot during the session. Clothing should cover all areas that the harness will cover to avoid skin irritation or chafing from the rough fabric of the harness during movement.

The client may engage in step training either in shoes or in stocking feet. Training the client in stocking feet or slippers maximizes afferent input to the soles of the feet, providing an important sensory cue for locomotion. Occasionally, shoes and socks are removed during brief periods of step training. This allows the trainers to observe and facilitate the client's foot and ankle position during the gait cycle and to aid in enhancing sensory cues from the sole of the foot, most likely cutaneous. The trainers and client should inspect the skin of the feet regularly, especially the toes, during and after training for any signs of irritation. If inflammation or abrasions occur, the areas should be immediately padded or protected with tape, or the client should wear shoes. If the client needs to wear foot protection, thin, lightweight shoes serve as the best footwear for training. Thick-soled and/or highly cushioned shoes should be avoided as they restrict afferent input to the sole of the foot. Heavy shoes may prevent independent swing action. High-top shoes interfere with appropriate hand placements and may restrict the range of motion of the ankle, altering intra-limb joint kinematics of the hip and knee. Braces are not used during step training as they also may alter limb kinematics and critical sensory input.

Applying the Harness

The support apparatus consists of two parts: the harness vest and the pelvic belt. Correct fit is essential for success in training. If the apparatus slips out of place, the trainer should stop the session and readjust the fit before proceeding. Correct harness fit should be established on the first training day to maximize comfort and to expedite preparation for the rest of the training sessions. Initially, the harness vest and pelvic belt should be

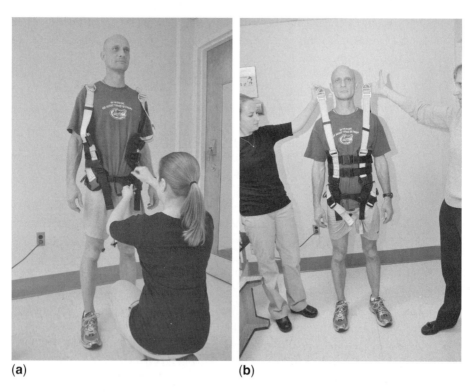

(a)   **(b)**

FIG 4-1 a, b. Harness placement (Roberson Harness, Henderson, NV) with client in standing position.

separate, with all buckles and straps disconnected. The support apparatus should be fitted to the client while he or she is in a standing position (Fig. 4-1a and 4-1b). When this is not possible, the support apparatus should be fitted to the client while he or she is lying on a table or mat. The harness vest and pelvic belt are placed on the mat separately and the client should lie on top of them in the approximate position for proper fit. The trainers can roll the client from side to side to adjust the position of the harness and to secure buckles and straps.

Pelvic Belt Placement

The pelvic belt is applied to the client first (Fig. 4-2a and 4-2b). Placement should be symmetrical, with support distributed evenly across the pelvis without limiting

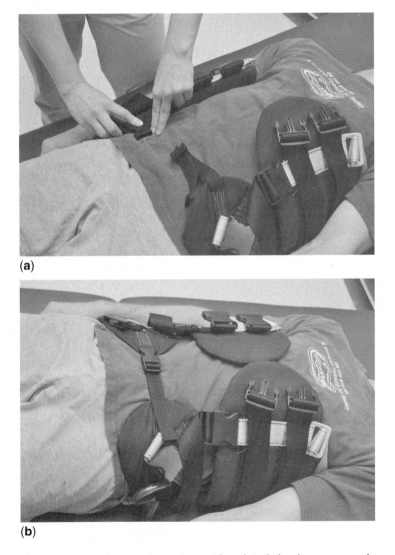

(a)

(b)

FIG 4-2 a, b. Harness application in supine with pelvic belt placement at the anterior iliac spine.

hip extension. The pelvic belt straps must be very tight so that most of the weight is supported at the pelvis and not around the ribs. The pelvic belt should firmly grip the pelvis by placement just under the anterior superior iliac spines.

Harness Vest Placement

The harness vest is applied to the client next; it should firmly grip the rib cage (Fig. 4-3). The lower trunk strap should be placed just underneath the lower rib cage. Dycem or a thin material with friction can be used between the client's chest and the vest to prevent slippage. The upper strap is placed just below the breasts. It is important to snug the lower strap so the harness vest firmly grips the client below the ribcage. The upper strap can be loosened slightly or padding added inside the vest if the client is uncomfortable. Next, the anterior and posterior harness vest straps are tightened to achieve the tightest fit that does not impede respiration.

Leg Strap Placement

Leg straps are applied one at a time (Fig. 4-4a and 4-4b). In men, the trainer should assist or have the client move his genitals away from the straps to avoid pinching. The trainer should check carefully after straps are snug to see that genitals are clear of the straps. Lycra, Spandex, Neoprene sleeves, or gel pads can be used on the straps in the groin area to minimize friction and rubbing. Padding may also be available to cover the leg straps. If the client uses an indwelling or condom catheter and leg bag, the trainer should make sure that the leg straps do not pinch the hose or impede the flow. The hose should move horizontally across the superior anterior thigh and down along the lateral aspect of the thigh. The trainer should check to make sure there are no kinks or folds in the hose, and ensure that urine is flowing into the bag. After several minutes of stepping, the leg bag and hose should be rechecked.

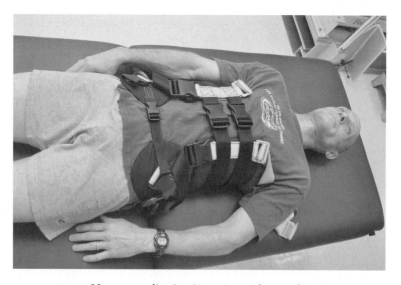

FIG 4-3 Harness application in supine with vest placement.

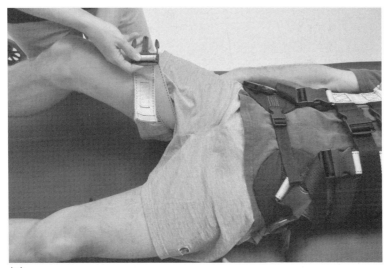

(a)

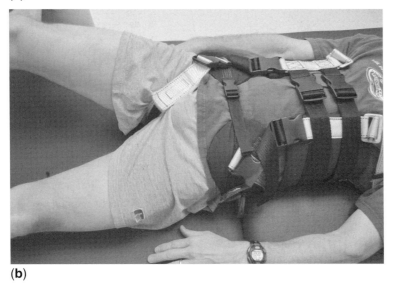

(b)

FIG 4-4 a, b. Leg strap placement.

Final Adjustments and Troubleshooting Harness Fit

One trainer holds the harness vest and another trainer holds the pelvic belt while a third trainer tightens the four vertical connector straps (two in front and two in back) that hold the vest and belt together. If one trainer is fitting the harness, the harness vest and pelvic bands must remain in position while the four vertical connector straps are tightened. Once the pelvis belt, harness vest, and straps are applied, final adjustments are made to ensure proper fit and to prevent slippage during step training. Harness fit should be checked when the client is seated in an erect posture.

The location of the clip over the shoulder can influence trunk alignment. The clips are placed over the midpoint of the shoulders initially, regardless of whether the clip is at

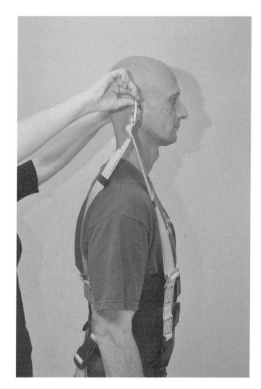

FIG 4-5 Alignment of the clip at mid-shoulder position. If applied in sitting, recheck in standing position.

the shoulder or above the shoulder (Fig. 4-5). If the clip is placed anterior to the shoulder midline, a plumb line falling from the overhead support cable through the harness straps will fall anterior to the trunk (Fig. 4-6). This will minimize trunk flexion and provide a more erect trunk posture. While this position may seem advantageous for a client who is unable to maintain an upright trunk, continued and prolonged use of this technique will not promote learning of trunk and postural control. Though the position affords alignment, the client must learn the ability to control an upright trunk position. In comparison, if the clip is placed posterior to the shoulder midline, the plumb line falls posterior to the trunk, promoting trunk flexion. Improper harness fit can affect the quality of the stepping by putting the client at a kinematic disadvantage. This includes causing trunk flexion or hyperextension, excess trunk lateral movement, and hip extension limitation. Table 4-1 lists some common harness fit problems and solutions.

System Requirements

Client safety and trainer ergonomics are important considerations when choosing a BWST system. A proper BWST system is critical for safe training of the client (Fig. 4-7). The system should allow for comfortable trainer positioning (e.g., ergonomic seating) with easy access to the client's hips and legs. Support of the trainer's back and a foot/leg support for stabilization during training are necessary. Seat adjustability for optimal

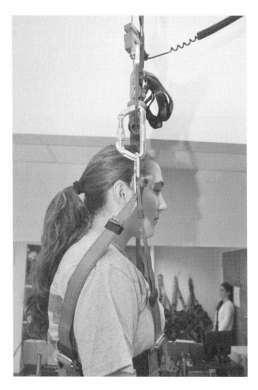

FIG 4-6 Alignment of the clip anterior to the shoulder position.

trainer positioning will enhance the effectiveness of the training and the long-term health of each trainer. The support system should allow for safe stepping and should prevent falls with a provision for releasing the client from the support quickly if needed. Thus, the training system must have a "safety" mechanism that allows the client the ability to stumble, trip, or misstep during walking, while further allowing him or her to self-correct his or her step and balance to prevent a fall. A backup overhead safety cable to the BWS system is adjusted to prevent a fall to the floor during training.

A feedback system indicating the immediate load during all standing or stepping activities on the treadmill is optimal because it provides online information for establishing training goals and for monitoring the client's response. A dynamic feedback system that constantly adjusts the BWS to maintain continuous support and that also allows the typical sinusoidal pattern of the body's center of mass during walking will optimize the retraining of the nervous system for overground walking. As this pattern is consistent with normal walking, it is an important component of the ensemble of sensory information provided by the training experience to generate an appropriate stepping pattern. This element of the BWS system may be even more important for clients with limited activation of the trunk and leg musculature to control the forces upon the limbs and body during weight transitions and loading while walking. The treadmill should also have variable controls, with the ability to slowly increase speed and to start immediately at a given speed.

A bungee system provides extra stability in clients with challenging trunk, pelvis, and leg activity affecting the ability to achieve an upright posture and body position.

TABLE 4-1 **Some Common Harness Fit Problems and Solutions**

Improper Harness Fit	Resulting Problem	Solution
Harness vest tilted posteriorly (higher in front) or anteriorly (higher in back)	If harness is posteriorly tilted, it can cause trunk hyperextension If harness is anteriorly tilted, it can cause trunk flexion.	Loosen the back vertical connector straps between the pelvic belt and the vest and tighten the front connector straps. Adjust the shoulder straps so that the clips are midline over the shoulders. Loosen the front vertical connector straps between the pelvic belt and the vest and tighten the back connector straps. Adjust the shoulder straps so that the clips are midline over the shoulders.
Pelvic belt posteriorly tilted	Limits hip extension and causes client to "sit" in the harness.	Loosen leg straps and front vertical connector straps. Tilt the pelvic belt so that the front is lower and the belt fits straight. Tighten the back vertical connector straps and the leg straps.
Harness straps not snug against shoulder	Excess trunk lateral movement	Tighten the front and back shoulder straps so that the clips are snug against the shoulders.
Pelvic Belt too low on buttocks	Limits hip extension	Loosen the leg straps and raise the pelvic belt to the appropriate place. Tighten the leg straps and the vertical connector straps between the vest and pelvic belt.

The bungees may be placed from each upright support at the front corners of the BWST at the pelvic band level using connectors (Fig. 4-8a). The bungees cross in front of the client and hook onto the pelvic band. This position may permit better pelvic and trunk upright alignment. Bungees may also be used only behind the client as a counterforce to maintain body alignment with the overhead BWS system (Fig. 4-8b). If used, the bungee system should be removed as quickly as possible during the retraining process; this should occur before changing other parameters such as load or speed.

Trainers should continually evaluate the options available on the market. Access to the BWST via a wheelchair ramp and also stairs allows access for wheelchair users and clients who walk. Negotiation of the ramp or stairs may be practiced with a client as she or he begins and ends the step training session on the treadmill.

Positioning Client on Treadmill with Body Weight Support

Four trainers are needed to position the client on the BWST. Leg trainers should be in their seats on the sides of the treadmill before the client is brought onto the treadmill belt in a wheelchair. The hip trainer is responsible for pushing the client in a wheelchair up the ramp and onto the treadmill belt (Fig. 4-9a). There should always be a trainer behind

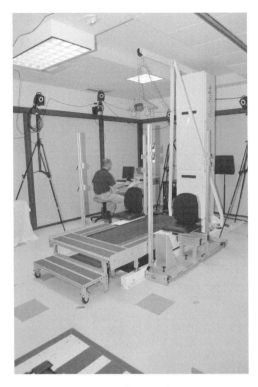

FIG 4-7 A body weight support system (Therastride, Innoventor, St. Louis, MO) with overhead safety, treadmill, and ergonomic seating system for the leg trainers with back and leg/foot support.

the wheelchair as a safety precaution. The wheelchair is positioned so that the client's feet are directly under the BWS cable and hanger and are placed in a position ready to bear weight (Fig. 4-9b). Removable or swing-away leg/foot rests on the wheelchair make positioning the legs for weight-bearing easier. When coming from sit-to-stand from a rigid front-end wheelchair, the client's feet may have to be placed forward, requiring greater physical assistance to transition weight from the seat to the legs. A trainer in front of the wheelchair attaches the overhead BWS cable and the harness to the overhead hanger (Fig. 4-9b). With the leg trainers in place, a trainer standing in front of the client, and a trainer guarding the client from behind, the is increased (approximately 50% to 60%) to assist in the transition from sit-to-stand and to achieve standing (Fig. 4-9c and 4-9d).

Once the client is standing, the leg trainers monitor and assist in knee extension. A trainer standing in front of the client places the additional safety into place (Fig. 4-9e). The length is adjusted to allow the client to fall between 2 and 4 inches before this backup safety "catches" the client. The trainer behind the client may now remove the chair (Fig. 4-9f). A trainer steps in behind the client and becomes the hip trainer. Clients may already be standing or walking overground prior to initiating Locomotor Training. If so, the client may be able to either walk up an incline or step up several steps to the BWST system. The trainer should continuously assess the client's comfort level

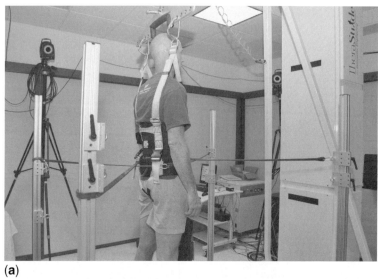

(a)

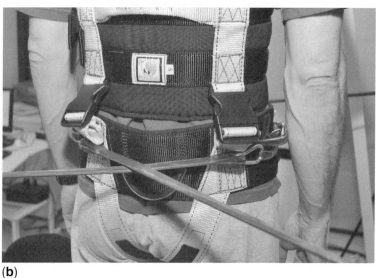

(b)

FIG 4-8 **a, b**. Bungee system for extra stability.

and monitor heart rate and blood pressure, as appropriate. If the client reports dizziness, the trainer should try stepping or marching right away, as this may alleviate orthostatic hypotension.

Client and Trainer Positions During Standing

During standing, the client and the trainers (physical therapists and trainers) work together to establish and maintain a properly aligned and erect posture (Fig. 4-10). Proper alignment enables the client to optimize the sensory cues and kinematics needed for

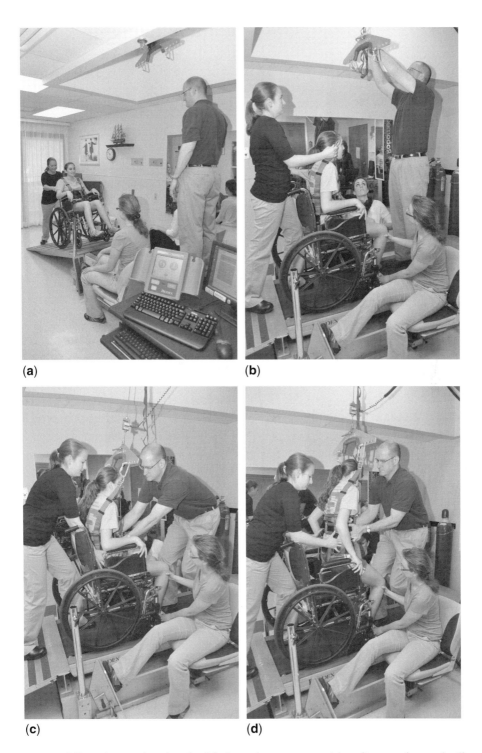

(a)   (b)

(c)   (d)

FIG 4-9 a. Hip trainer pushes the wheelchair up the ramp to position client on the treadmill. Leg trainers are ready and seated by the treadmill. **b.** The wheelchair is positioned so that the client's feet are directly under the body weight support cable and hanger. A trainer positioned in front of the wheelchair assists with attaching the overhead hanger to the harness.

(*Continues*)

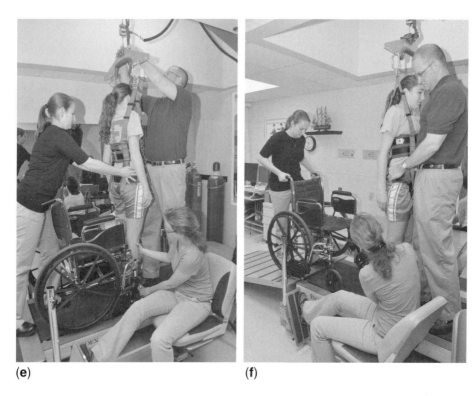

(e)   **(f)**

FIG 4-9 (continued)   **c, d.** The two trainers assist the client from sit-to-stand with use of the body weight support while the leg trainers monitor and assist with leg position. **e.** Once the client is in standing position, the leg trainers monitor leg position and the trainer in front attaches and adjusts the body weight support safety. **f.** The trainer behind then removes the wheelchair and either steps in or another trainer steps in as the hip trainer.

locomotion. Three trainers may be needed to assist the client during standing. The hip trainer straddles the treadmill belt and is positioned behind the client. The leg trainer or trainers sit on either side of the treadmill belt next to a leg.

Client Position

The client should maintain erect posture during stand training. A mirror may be placed in front of the client and another to the side of the client to provide feedback to the client and trainers concerning alignment. Align head, shoulders, hips, and feet directly under the support cable (erect posture) and maintain alignment continuously during standing. The knees should remain in extension while avoiding hyperextension. The ankles should be maintained in neutral position, avoiding excessive inversion or eversion. The heels should be placed firmly on the treadmill surface (Fig. 4-11).

Hip Trainer

The hip trainer is primarily responsible for establishing and maintaining proper client position and alignment. This trainer straddles the treadmill behind the client and firmly

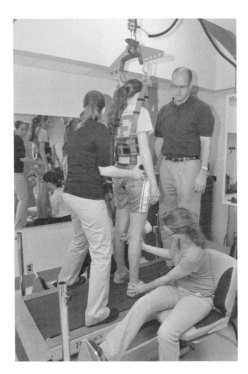

FIG 4-10 Client and trainers work together to establish proper alignment and erect posture on the treadmill with body weight support.

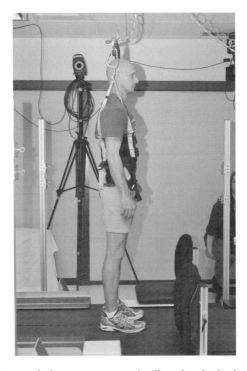

FIG 4-11 Client position and alignment on treadmill under the body weight support cable and hanger.

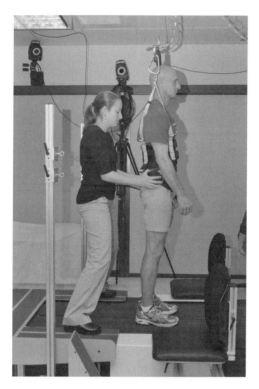

FIG 4-12 Hip trainer position.

grasps the pelvis and/or trunk area of the harness (Fig. 4-12). The trainer's knees and elbows should be flexed to allow him or her to maintain balance and move with the client and provides assistance (such as assisting with pelvic rotation) only when necessary. The trainer should continually cue the client verbally to encourage independence in head, shoulder, trunk, and pelvis positions. The hip trainer is also in an optimal position to monitor the client's response to the intervention and level of comfort, and to provide verbal cueing, using the mirror to assess the client's response.

Leg Trainers

The leg trainers are positioned on the sides of and facing the opposite direction of the client. Each trainer's feet are planted firmly on the floor or braced on the supports. The shoulders of the trainer should be in front of the client's knee, and when his or her hands are placed below the client's knee during standing, the trainer's elbow is at a 90-degree bend. This mid-position will ensure that the trainer can promote full hip extension during the stance phase and also assist in foot placement during the transition from swing to stance (i.e., foot contact; Fig. 4-13). In addition, the trainer is able to move the seat inward or outward from the treadmill to accommodate the size of his or her arm and trunk. The trainer should maintain his or her back in contact with the support to promote an upright trunk and a stable position from which to facilitate the client's leg

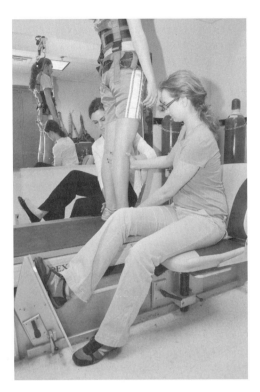

FIG 4-13 Leg trainer position.

pattern or posture during training. A leg support may also be used to further provide stability for the trainer's position. The support is adjustable to allow flexion of the trainer's leg.

Correct placement of the trainer's hands is critical to optimize retraining of the client's nervous system. Specific sensory cues resulting from proper hand placement stimulate specific motor output. Hand placement can facilitate activation of standing through the sensory and motor pathways. When assisting with a movement, the trainer should always aim to facilitate the movement as it would normally be performed. The leg trainer provides assistance only when necessary to facilitate independence in the legs. The trainer asks the client first to move and then assesses whether the movement kinematics and timing were appropriate. If appropriate, then no assistance is provided. If the movement is not typical or is slow, then manual facilitation may be provided to promote the movement. This process is repeated time and again as the therapist continually monitors client advancement in skill and independence of movement before facilitating the movement.

- Placing the hands on the extensor tendons stimulates afferent input that facilitates an extensor motor response. To promote extension, hands should be placed on the patellar (quadriceps) and Achilles tendons (Fig. 4-14). The hand should not be placed over the patella. Placement on the patellar tendon thus occurs during the transition from swing to stance and during the stance phase of gait, as needed.

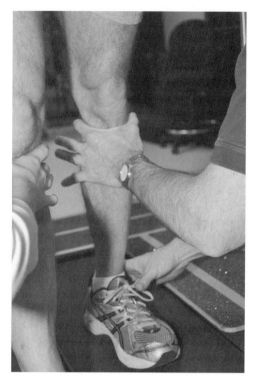

FIG 4-14 Leg trainer hand placement for promoting extension.

- Placing the hands on the flexor tendons stimulates afferent input that facilitates a flexor motor response. To promote flexion, the hands should be placed on the hamstrings and tibialis anterior tendons (Fig. 4-15). Placement is predominantly on the medial hamstrings using the standard hand placement for knee control. Hand placement is located on the lateral hamstrings using the alternate hand hold to emphasize foot and ankle control. The hamstrings are cued above the popliteal fossa (posterior knee crease). The tibialis anterior is cued via light to medium pressure on the tendon. Placement of the hands on the hamstrings and tibialis anterior tendons occurs during the transition from stance to swing and during the swing phase of gait, as needed.

Client and Trainer Positions During Stepping

During stepping, the trainers must establish and maintain a properly aligned and erect posture and proper leg kinematics. Proper alignment positions the client to optimize the sensory cues and kinematics needed for locomotion. Proper leg kinematics are achieved with extension during stance and flexion of the hip, knee, and ankle during swing.

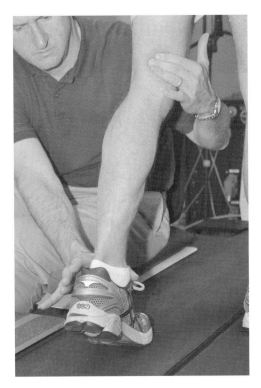

FIG 4-15 Leg trainer hand placement for promoting flexion.

Client Position

The client should maintain erect posture during step training. Head, shoulders, hips, and feet should be aligned directly under the support cable (erect posture), and alignment should be maintainted continuously during stepping. During stance, the hip should move through extension and the knees should remain in extension, while avoiding hyperextension. The ankles should be maintained in neutral position, avoiding excessive inversion or eversion, and the heels should be placed firmly on the treadmill surface. At toe-off or during the transition from stance to swing, the stance-limb hip has reached maximal extension, the knee is in extension, and the ankle has progressed from neutral to dorsiflexion to plantarflexion. Push-off occurs with the hip in extension and the ankle in plantarflexion. As the body weight then shifts from the stance limb forward to the opposite limb (now loading), the leg begins to flex at the hip, knee, and ankle into the swing phase. During swing, the hips and knees should move through flexion while avoiding excessive abduction/adduction and internal/external hip rotation. The ankles should dorsiflex while avoiding excessive inversion or eversion. As the limb advances during swing, the hip flexes and the knee joint extends to bring the foot forward of the knee and ready for contact with the ground. The foot should contact the ground with a heel strike and should be positioned in slight dorsiflexion and the knee in slight flexion.

Hip Trainer

The hip trainer is responsible for establishing and maintaining proper client position and alignment and control of the pelvis during stepping. Rotation of the pelvis is coordinated with leg movement during stepping, and forward weight shift occurs associated with a single step or during a transition from the swing to stance phase of gait. Align the head, shoulders, hips, and feet directly under the support cable (erect posture) and maintain alignment continuously during stepping. The trainer should stand approximately 20 cm (8 inches) or the length of the trainer's forearm behind the client and firmly grasp the harness handles. There are three possible hand positions, and the choice of position may depend upon the particular goal or training focus for the hip trainer:

- Rear handle of vest and lateral handle of pelvic band (Fig. 4-16a): This hand hold provides control of the upright posture and lateral stabilization of the pelvis. This may be selected for asymmetry at the pelvis or trunk.
- Rear handle of vest and rear handle of pelvic band (Fig. 4-16b and 4-16c). This hand hold maximizes the assistance provided to establish an upright trunk posture over the pelvis and feet.
- Both lateral handles of pelvic band (Fig. 4-16d): This position provides the greatest support to promote hip rotation. With no hand hold on the vest, the trunk is typically exhibiting good upright posture and control.

During the stance phase, the trainer will assist the client in rotating the pelvis from front to back (Fig. 4-17a). During the stance-to-swing transition, the trainer will assist the client with weight shift to the other leg, and during the swing phase, the trainer will assist the client in rotating the pelvis back to front and prevent the hip from dropping (Fig. 4-17b). During the swing-to-stance transition, the trainer will assist with weight shift onto the stance leg (Fig. 4-17c). The trainer limits the pelvis from tilting anteriorly, posteriorly, and laterally while assisting rotation of the pelvis along the longitudinal axis during stepping. To do this, trainers should keep their arms rigid and rotate their own body simultaneously with the client. Trainers can place their elbows against their own body to help keep their arms rigid. If less assistance is needed, the trainer can hold the handles of the pelvic band to provide corrections. The client should not be allowed to lean back on the trainer; the only contact between the trainer and client should be with the trainer's hands. The trainer should be continuously giving verbal cues to the client to encourage independent head, shoulder, trunk, and pelvis movements.

Leg Trainers

The leg trainers are primarily responsible for assisting the client with leg movement. In the standard hand placement ("knee control" is emphasized), the inside, upper hand assists with the knee and is critical for the facilitation of flexion and extension. The outside, lower hand assists at the ankle and is used only to assist toe clearance at lift-off ("toe-off") and foot placement at initial contact ("heel strike"). Correct placement of

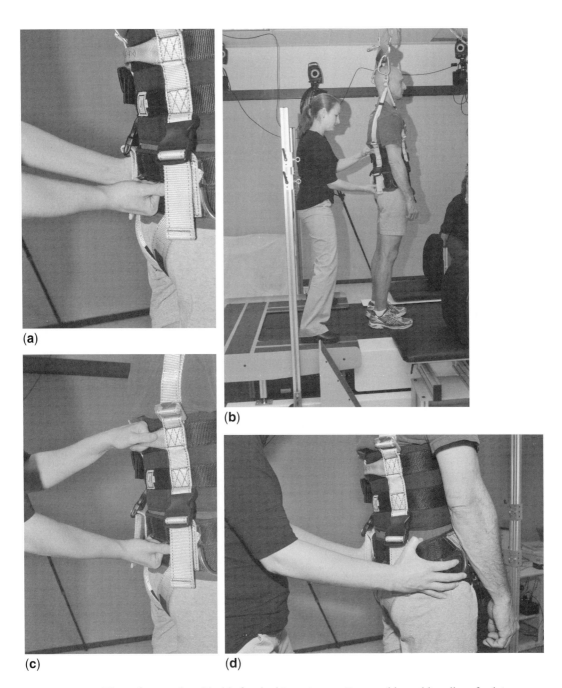

(a)

(b)

(c)

(d)

FIG 4-16 Three alternate hand holds for the hip trainer. **a.** Rear and lateral handles of pelvic band. **b, c.** Rear handle of vest and rear handle of pelvic band. **d.** Both lateral handles of pelvic band.

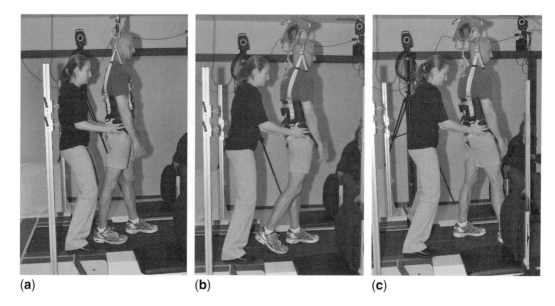

(a)   (b)   (c)

FIG 4-17 Hip trainer role during stepping. **a.** Weight-bearing with right hip and knee in extension in stride position. Pelvis is rotated slightly backward and downward. **b.** Weight shift forward onto left leg. **c.** Swing-to-stand transition of the right leg. Pelvis rotates slightly forward and upward.

the trainer's hands is critical to optimize retraining of the client's nervous system. Hand placement facilitates activation of stepping through the sensory and motor neural connections. Specific sensory cues resulting from proper hand placement stimulate specific motor output. The leg trainers provide assistance only when necessary to facilitate and promote muscle activation in the legs and proper alignment.

- Placing the hands on the extensor surface during stance stimulates extensor sensory neurons and facilitates an extensor motor response.
- Placing the hands on the flexor surface during swing stimulates flexor sensory neurons and facilitates a flexor motor response.

During the stance phase, the trainer assists with knee extension (Fig. 4-18a) by gently pushing with the upper hand on the proximal tibia at the patellar tendon. The trainer should avoid applying too much force and locking the knee in extension. The dorsum of the foot is stabilized to control eversion/inversion with the lower hand.

During the stance-to-swing transition, the trainer facilitates swing by pressing on the medial hamstrings, with two fingers only. The trainer pushes up on the ankle at the tibialis anterior tendon to provide a counter-force and assist toe clearance (Fig. 4-18b). *Note: Trainers should not wear jewelry because it can scratch the client or the other trainers.*

During swing, the trainer guides the knee through using only forward pressure at the medial hamstring (Fig. 4-18c). The trainer should avoid grabbing the calf. The trainer

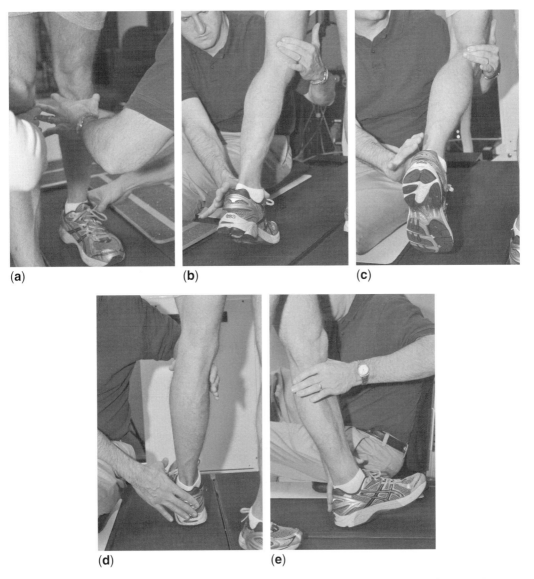

(a) **(b)** **(c)**

(d) **(e)**

FIG 4-18 Leg trainer standard hand positions to facilitate stepping (knee control position). Note that jewelry such as rings and watches should not be worn during training on the treadmill.

Inside Upper Hand Placement

a. Stance phase—extension of hip and knee. Place web of hand at anterior, proximal tibia, just below the patella. Provide just enough force to achieve knee extension without hyperextension.

b. Stance-to-swing phase—transition from extension to flexion of hip and knee. Rotate hand from the anterior tibia to the medial hamstring tendon (medially and upwardly).

c. Swing phase—flexion of hip and knee. Move arm backwards (into extension) through mid-swing. Guide knee through swing. Rotate hand back to the front of the knee at terminal swing.

(Continues)

should avoid rotating and pulling the knee toward himself or herself. The trainer should keep the elbow of his or her upper hand up.

During the swing-to-stance transition, the trainer gently pushes on the proximal tibia at the patellar tendon while also pushing on the back of the ankle (Fig. 4-18d and 4-18e). This produces a counter-force to the push with the upper hand to achieve knee extension.

Alternate Hand Placements

In certain circumstances, alternate hand placements are desirable. When a client requires greater assistance at the knee during the transition from swing to stance (loading) or during the support phase to promote upright support, the standard hand hold (emphasis on knee control) is used. When a client requires greater facilitation and assistance at the ankle or foot to activate and achieve good limb kinematics during stepping and needs minimal assistance at the knee, the reverse hand placement (or "ankle control") is chosen. This may also be used when stepping a client without shoes or socks.

Reverse Hand Placement

A reverse hand placement ("ankle control" emphasis) is used if foot inversion/plantarflexion is a problem during the swing or stance phases and the client does not need help with knee extension. In this instance, independent control of the knee has been achieved while facilitation of the ankle is still necessary. It is also helpful if the client is toe dragging and/or placing the foot at or near the midline (hip adduction). Reverse hand placement puts the trainer at a mechanical disadvantage for assisting with knee extension during stance. Therefore, it should not be used when considerable help with knee extension is needed. In reverse hand placement ("ankle control"), the outside hand is positioned at the knee (outside, upper hand placement) and the inside hand is positioned at the foot

---

FIG 4-18 (continued)

d, e. Swing-to-stance phase—transition from flexion to extension of hip and knee. Finish rotating hand to front of the knee. Provide just enough force to the anterior, proximal tibia so the knee is extended at initial contact. Avoid pushing on the patella.

Outside Lower Hand Placement

a. Stance phase—extension of hip and knee. Stabilize dorsum of foot if client tends to evert or invert.

b. Stance-to-swing phase—transition from extension to flexion of hip and knee. Assist foot clearance at lift-off by gently pushing upward at the anterior surface of the ankle.

c. Swing phase—flexion of hip and knee. Move arm backwards (into extension) through mid-swing. Guide knee through swing. Avoid contacting the posterior ankle (Achilles tendon) during mid-swing.

d, e. Swing-to-stance phase—transition from flexion to extension of hip and knee. Rotate the fingers to the back of the heel at the end of swing and assist the foot through to initial contact.

(inside, lower hand placement; Fig. 4-19a). The inside, lower hand is placed on the dorsum of the foot (with web space at the tibialis tendon; Fig. 4-19b) rather than at the ankle to assist with foot lift-off and initial contact (Fig. 4-19c). The trainer should avoid touching or grasping the plantar surface of the foot, as this can elicit extension of the ankle, knee, and hip or trigger clonus or spasm in the limb. The outside, upper hand is placed at the posterior knee to assist with knee flexion (Fig. 4-19d). The trainer should avoid grabbing the calf.

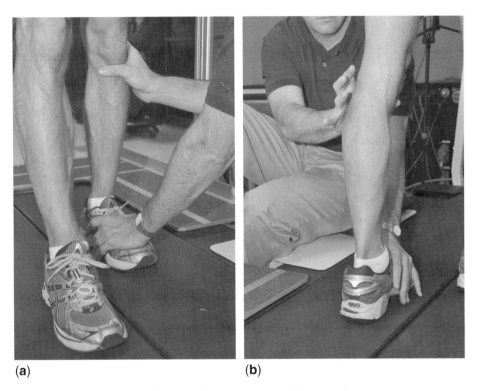

(a)   **(b)**

FIG 4-19 Leg trainer alternate hand position (reverse or ankle control).
Outside Upper Hand Placement
a. Stance phase—extension of hip and knee. Place thumb at anterior, proximal tibia, just below the patella. Provide enough force to achieve knee extension.
b. Stance-to-swing phase—transition from extension to flexion of hip and knee. Rotate hand from the anterior tibia to the lateral hamstring tendon (laterally and upwardly).
c. Swing phase—flexion of hip and knee. Move arm across own chest through mid-swing. Guide knee through swing. Rotate hand back to the front of the knee at terminal swing.
d. Swing-to-stance phase—transition from flexion to extension of hip and knee. Finish rotating hand to front of the knee. Provide just enough force to the anterior, proximal tibia so the knee is extended at initial contact. Avoid pushing on the patella.

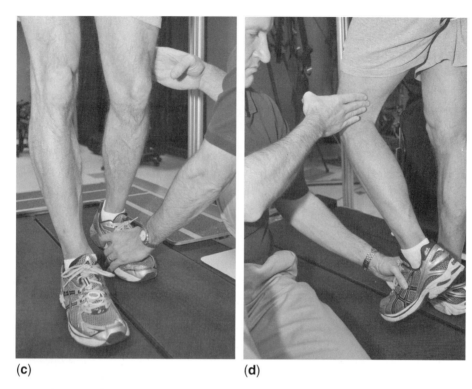

(c)   **(d)**

FIG 4-19 (continued)

Inside Lower Hand Placement

a. Stance phase—extension of hip and knee. Stabilize dorsum of foot if client tends to evert or invert.

b. Stance-to-swing phase—transition from extension to flexion of hip and knee. Assist foot clearance at lift-off by gently lifting upward on the dorsum of the foot and pushing backward.

c. Swing phase—flexion of hip and knee. Move arm backwards (into extension) through mid-swing. Control inversion and eversion while keeping hand on dorsum of the foot. Do not touch plantar surface of foot.

d. Swing-to-stance phase—transition from flexion to extension of hip and knee. Guide foot to initial contact and prevent inversion and eversion. Assist with dorsiflexion and heel contact if needed.

Modified Standard Hand Placement

A modified standard hand placement (outside, lower hand only) is used if foot inversion or eversion is a problem and the client needs assistance with knee extension. It is also helpful if the client is toe dragging and/or placing the foot at or crossing the midline (hip adduction). Modified standard hand placement puts the trainer at more of a mechanical disadvantage compared to the reverse hand placement for controlling inversion/eversion and toe clearance. Therefore, this technique should be used only when knee extension must be controlled as well as ankle inversion/eversion. In the modified standard hand placement, the inside, upper hand position remains the same as in the standard, but the

TABLE 4-2 Trainer Positions, Hand Placement, and Techniques: Troubleshooting

Challenge	Potential Sources	Solutions
Trainer is rapidly fatiguing.	• Trainer is over-assisting the client. • Trainer is too tense and may be holding the leg or hip rigidly. • Trainer is using incorrect or counterproductive techniques.	• Guide, but don't force the legs. These are facilitation techniques, not dependent, full-assistive techniques. • The trainer should relax and avoid tensing the jaw and other muscles not involved in the activity; review proper body alignment. • Review hand placements and locomotor training techniques. • The trainer needs to communicate when s/he is tired. Brief rests are reasonable when developing skills for locomotor training. • Rotation of trainers within a session to provide relief when fatigued.
Leg trainer seems to be working too hard, (e.g., rocking back and forth in the seat).	• Leg trainer is seated too far away from the subject. • Leg trainer is flexing and extending trunk for force production. • Client's hips are too far back on the treadmill.	• The trainer should remain directly adjacent to the treadmill belt. • Gauge trainer distance from the standing client. The upper arm (at tibia) and lower arm (at ankle) should be comfortably flexed with room for arm extension. • Maintain erect, seated posture and extend and flex the arms, not the trunk. • Cue the hip trainer to bring the hips forward on the treadmill *slowly* across a few steps.
Hip trainer seems to be working too hard.	• Hand-grip/position may be inappropriate for that client. • Gripping the harness straps too hard. • Hip trainer is standing too far away from or too close to the subject. • Hip trainer is attempting to control too much movement. • Hip trainer is fighting against the client's natural hip rotation.	• Use alternate hand grips on the harness. • Relax hand grip on straps. • Evaluate if hip trainer is constantly lifting up on the harness. Client weight should be absorbed through the client's legs, not the hip trainer. • The hip trainer should remain about forearm length away from the client. • Allow natural rotation of the client's hips to flow with the legs, providing corrections only as needed. • Hip trainer should keep knees slightly bent.

(continues)

Challenge	Potential Sources	Solutions
Upper hand is slipping onto patella.	• Leg trainer is pushing up. • Leg trainer is grabbing leg during swing. • Leg trainer is not rotating hand during swing to stance transition.	• Keep web space of upper hand on the anterior tibia during swing to stance. • Review proper hand placements. • Record a video and go back to watch for mistakes • Timing of transitions improves with practice
Leg trainer is providing too much assistance at the ankle.	• Lower hand is grasping circumferentially around the ankle, squeezing the Achilles tendon.	• Place the hand on only one surface of the ankle at a time; anteriorly to aid with client ankle flexion during stance to swing and posteriorly to aid in client ankle extension during swing to stance. • Maintain a relatively open hand, to avoid squeezing or grasping the ankle tightly with the fingers.
Client's body alignment is upright but at a slight diagonal angle.	• Client is not directly underneath BWS pulley. • Harness straps have slipped and are uneven. • Client is directly underneath the pulley but hips are anteriorly tilted.	• Check that the pulley cable is vertical. • Check client from all sides to ensure that his/her center of gravity is directly below the pulley. • During standing, check that the client's feet are in line with the knees and hips (proper body alignment). • Adjust harness straps as needed. • Hip trainer should apply a posterior tilt to the hips.
Leg trainer hand placement is not coordinated within stance to swing phase of step cycle.	• Upper hand is at the anterior side of the proximal tibia during client's knee flexion. • Leg trainer is not rotating hand. • Upper hand is on the hamstring tendon or the medial side of the knee during client's knee extension. • Timing of hand rotation is off.	• Avoid placing the upper hand on the anterior surface during stance to swing phase. The trainer needs to rotate the hand from the anterior tibia to the hamstring tendon (initiating hamstring contraction and knee flexion) during the stance to swing phase. • Avoid placing the upper hand on the posterior surface during swing to stance phase. The trainer needs to rotate the hand back to the front of the knee during the swing to stance phase. • Practice coordination. • Have a sidelined person/treadmill operator cue trainer's hand placement.

TABLE 4.2 *(Continued)*

Challenge	Potential Sources	Solutions
During swing, hip and knee flexion is inhibited or slowed.	• The upper hand is pushing on the anterior surface of the tibia. • The lower hand is resisting the limb as it moves forward through flexion. • Lower hand is grasping the Achilles tendon.	• Upper hand should not contact the anterior surface of the tibia during swing. • Avoid holding the ankle with the lower hand and adding resistance to the forward motion of the ankle. The hands should facilitate motor activation, not impede it. • The trainer needs to develop hand coordination in the stance to swing transition. • Avoid grabbing the Achilles tendon. Keep an open lower hand (not clenched).
	• Rotation at hips is not synchronized. • Leg trainer is not contacting the hamstring tendon.	• Hip trainer may need to allow some rotation at a similar movement rate of the legs. • Hip trainer may need to prevent the hip from dropping by slightly holding-up on the swing side. • Upper hand should reach up to the hamstring tendon during swing and avoid grabbing the calf.
During swing, hip and knee flexion are exaggerated or too rapid.	• The leg trainer is over-assisting the forward motion of the limb and exceeding normal limb excursion for swing. • The leg trainer is forcing the limb upward and forward through flexion.	• Guide and allow limb advancement to occur at client's self-generated pace as opposed to forcing the limb through the motion too strongly and rapidly. • Avoid pushing or pulling the limb. Too much assistance can shut down, rather than facilitate, motor activation. • Cue all trainers (legs and hip) to slow down and relax.
Client's entire body is swaying side to side.	• Hip trainer is bouncing left to right. • Hip trainer is allowing too much lateral movement.	• Cue the hip trainer to stay steady – do NOT bounce side to side. • Cue hip trainer to squeeze in to counterbalance the client's lateral movement on the swing side.

(continues)

Challenge	Potential Sources	Solutions
Client's trunk only is swaying side to side	• Hip trainer is allowing too much lateral movement. • Leg trainers are stepping too close to the midline. • Harness straps need to be adjusted	• Cue hip trainer to squeeze in to counterbalance the client's lateral movement on the swing side. • Cue the leg trainers to widen their stance. • Adjust the harness straps.
During stance, knee is not fully extended.	• The upper hand is on the posterior surface of the tibia, behind the knee. • Hand coordination within step cycle is off. • The upper hand is not applying enough assistance to achieve and hold extension through stance.	• The trainer needs to develop hand coordination in the stance to swing transition. • Prepare the limb for hip and knee extension during stance by making sure that the knee is fully extended upon initial contact (heel strike). • Apply enough force to provide an extensor torque that is adequate to keep the hip and knee extended during weight acceptance. Get a feel for the amount of force needed at the knee when the client is standing.
	• Extension at initial contact (heel strike) was not achieved due to lack of kick through with the lower hand. • Weight shift onto stance leg was too early at initial contact (heel strike) making it harder to extend the leg. • Hips are too far forward on the treadmill. • Client's center of mass has lowered.	• Stimulate the Achilles tendon in stance. • Make sure the timing/coordination between all trainers (including hip) is correct. • Cue the hip trainer to bring the hips forward on the treadmill *slowly* across a few steps. • Briefly increase BWS to re-establish good stepping.

TABLE 4.2 *(Continued)*

Challenge	Potential Sources	Solutions
Feet are pounding or slapping on initial contact (heel strike).	• Leg trainer is not guiding the foot down. • Hip trainer is shifting the weight too early on the stance limb. • Leg trainers are not holding extension long enough on the stance limb.	• Leg trainer should guide the foot down by pressing on the Achilles tendon. • Hip trainer should keep the weight on the stance limb until they hear the swing leg land. • Instruct leg trainers to hold extension until the swing leg lands.
Hip trainer loses balance on treadmill.	• When the client trip, the hip trainer is unbalanced and falls forward. • Hip trainer is leaning into client.	• Hip trainer's knees should be slightly bent to maintain center of gravity within base of support. • Hip trainer should check if they are too close or too far away from the client.
Client's trunk is flexed	• Harness straps have slipped and are too far from the client's shoulders. • Client is leaning forward. • Client may have high flexor activity and need more trunk and hip assistance.	• Adjust harness straps as needed. • Verbally cue client to stand tall and bring their trunk back. • Hip trainer should try different hand holds.
Trainers are unable to recover stepping after a trip.	• Trainers are not communicating with each other. • The client is too low to the ground to regain knee extension.	• Trainers should cue which leg to go first. • Hip trainer should lift up and back until leg trainers regain their footing. • Possibly increase the BWS.

lower hand is placed and stays on the dorsum of the foot rather than at the ankle to assist with toe-off and heel strike. The trainer should avoid touching or grasping the plantar surface of the foot, as this can elicit extension of the ankle, knee, and hip or trigger clonus or spasm in the limb. The trainer should also avoid lifting or pushing the foot in an upward direction, as this may provide an inappropriate loading signal during swing. The leg trainer may use a modified standard hand placement to protect the toes when assisting clients without shoes.

5

Basic Skills for Retraining the Nervous System

Chapter Outline

Chapter Objectives

The objectives of Chapter 5 are to:

1. State the four components of step training and the goals of each component.
2. Describe the important kinematic factors and spatial-temporal walking pattern during the four phases of stepping: stance phase, stance-to-swing phase, swing phase, and swing-to-stance phase.
3. Describe the proper coordination among trainers during the four phases of the step cycle.
4. State the appropriate stride length and cadence.
5. Describe client position during standing.
6. Describe client position during initiating stepping (upright posture, stance position, and weight shift).
7. Describe the roles of the client and each training team member.

Summary

Step training is an essential component of Locomotor Training, providing retraining of the nervous system to stand and walk. Physical therapists and rehabilitation technicians must be skillful trainers while applying the Locomotor Training principles and mastering the techniques presented in this chapter. Individual trainers' actions are linked among the three trainers and the operation of the body weight support on the treadmill (BWST) to provide smooth assistive efforts to optimize interlimb coordination of the client and retraining of his or her neuromuscular system for locomotion. Step training requires a team: the client, a team leader, at least one additional trainer, and the BWST operator. Two additional trainers may assist when needed. Effective training requires not only physical coordination among the trainers but also verbal coordination and direction of the training effort via established goals for each session.

Locomotor Training: The Step Training Component

Step training builds walking capacity by retraining the nervous system, while the primary goal of both overground assessments and community integration is to translate this capacity to walking and function at home and in the community. Limitations to independent walking are identified during overground assessment and community integration and are specifically targeted in the step training sessions. Recovering the neural capacity to overcome these limitations is addressed more effectively during step training on the treadmill since body weight load, treadmill speed, and manual facilitation are easily adjusted so the client can achieve optimal stepping and retraining of the neuromuscular system in a safe environment. Engaging the client in the training process, setting goals, and progression from the first day and throughout the sessions is critical. The client will have 22.5 hours beyond the therapy session in which to make decisions that support the Locomotor Training principles. Knowledge of the principles and how they are applied in everyday activities can increase the amount of practice, repetition, and experience afforded the client's neuromuscular system beyond the clinic-based session in ways that support recovery.

The step training component of Locomotor Training includes four areas of focus: step retraining, step adaptability, stand retraining, and stand adaptability conducted using BWST environment. This system allows the principles to be optimally applied using manual facilitation as needed. The goal of step training is to retrain individuals to stand and step by taking advantage of the intrinsic mechanisms of the nervous system that generate neuromuscular activity. The primary relearning of the nervous system occurs in the step training component and is termed "retraining." "Stand retraining" bouts can be used to increase weight-bearing, improve balance, and improve trunk and pelvis control in clients who are not standing independently. Promotion of independence, improvement of balance, and resolution of gait deviations also occur in this environment; this is termed "adaptability." The relative amount of time of a total step training session spent in retraining versus adaptability and stand versus step retraining depends upon the client's level of recovery. Thus, the emphasis on each component depends on the projected course of recovery and the client's abilities along that continuum. The emphasis on specific components changes as the client progresses and recovers. Guidelines for progression are addressed in Chapter 8.

Step Retraining

In step retraining, assistance by BWS, manual facilitation, hand placement, and verbal cues are used to generate the necessary sensory input for facilitating upright postural control and coordinated stepping at natural walking speeds (Fig. 5-1). Step retraining should occur as the first and last bout of every step training session and should represent 20 to 45 minutes of the session. There are several factors to consider as the trainers interact with each other to promote a coordinated stepping pattern. The client's posture should be upright with the head aligned over the shoulders, and the shoulders over the trunk, and the upper body should be in line with the pelvis and the legs (knees, ankles, and feet). The head and trunk should remain in this upright and extended (neutral) position throughout step retraining. The pelvis should avoid tilting in the anterior, posterior, or lateral directions. It should rotate around the client's longitudinal axis in a rhythmic manner. Pelvic rotation is essential to achieve and maintain adequate trunk alignment and hip extension. Pelvic rotation is done in combination with weight shifting as the client's body weight load transfers from one leg to another during stepping, and also with hip, knee, and ankle flexion and extension during stance and swing, respectively. Coordination of leg and hip trainers is important to achieve the best stepping pattern with symmetrical placement and, most importantly, the timing of the loading and unloading of the legs to facilitate optimal neural activity.

Initiation

Stepping is always initiated with the client in the stride position. This position optimizes the kinematics to provide the sensory cues known to initiate swing. Thus, the client begins with the hip extended and then unloads that leg rapidly by shifting the body

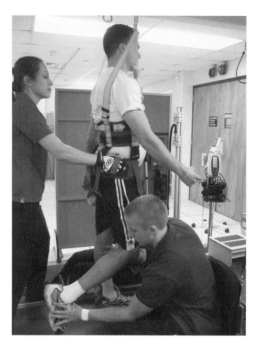

FIG 5-1 Step retraining.

weight to the other leg to generate flexion. The other leg, after accepting the load, moves backward, the hip and knee extend, the hip rotates slightly back, and the back leg is fully weight-bearing and now positioned with both hip and knee extended and the ankle dorsiflexed. If this pattern cannot be achieved independently, then the hip and leg trainer assist the client into the stride position and through the movement, providing assistance only when necessary. Verbal cues, hand placements, and tactile cues for facilitating these components of weight shift, leg flexion, leg extension, and then weight shift are provided. The trainer assisting the extended and loaded leg begins with his or her inside hand on the patellar tendon. As weight shift occurs from the extended and loaded leg to the other leg in the stride position, the trainer's hand placement switches to the flexor surfaces for the medial hamstring and tibialis anterior to promote leg flexion.

If the client can step into a stride position but uses a compensatory strategy to accomplish the movement; then the hip and leg trainer will instead assist the client through the correct, kinematic pattern consistent with the task. This facilitation and task specificity are repeated for each motor task that a client attempts to achieve. Thus, the reference for movement is the pre-injury movement pattern specific to the task. Trainers provide verbal instructions to the client before facilitating a movement. This gives the client the opportunity to independently move and to continually reassess his or her abilities relative to the goal of recovery.

Stance

During stance, the pelvis rotates posterior as the leg moves backward on the treadmill belt with full knee extension through mid-stance. The foot should remain firmly on the treadmill belt and avoid inversion/eversion. The trainer assists the client to achieve the stance phase only as needed.

Stance-to-Swing Transition

During the stance-to-swing transition, the client shifts his or her weight from the stance leg to the other leg at terminal stance. The process of initiating swing is also used during the stance-to-swing transition. Thus, unloading of the leg and sufficient hip extension should occur simultaneously at lift-off. Lift-off of the foot should occur only after the other foot is placed on the treadmill to achieve double-limb support. If assisting, the trainer should be careful not to lift the foot or release knee extension too early or the loading effect will be diminished. Foot placement is determined by considering stride length.

Stride length can vary according to the client's age, leg length, and stepping speed. Typically, the longer the client's legs, the greater the stride length needed for a step. Also, as treadmill speed increases, stride length increases. A practical guide in determining stride length is by placing the limb at both ends of the step cycle in relationship to the pelvis in a relatively fixed position with the head and trunk in line with the BWS cable. The trainer places the foot at initial contact and checks laterally that the knee and foot are in the proper position, with the knee extended and the foot in contact with the ground. The other foot is placed at terminal stance, just prior to lift-off, with the hip extended, knee beginning to flex, and toe ready to push off. Once an appropriate stride length is determined that allows weight shift with the proper pelvis and leg kinematics, markers are placed on the treadmill frame as an indicator of initial contact and lift-off locations. These may assist the leg trainers in maintaining an accurate stride length. Stride length may change based on the training variables, particularly speed, and with client independence.

Lift-off should occur at the same relative backward position on the treadmill belt for both legs to ensure proper stride length and avoid taking too long or too short steps. Coordination of leg trainers is important to achieve symmetrical gait when assistance is needed. Trainers simultaneously stimulate the medial hamstring tendon (to initiate knee flexion) with the upper hand and gently assist the ankle at the tibialis anterior with the lower hand to initiate swing. Trainers should ensure that the toe does not drag on the treadmill during initial swing by moving the ankle upward until knee flexion allows toe clearance. Trainers should avoid over-stimulation, which can result in excessive knee flexion. The tibialis anterior tendon is stimulated with pressure if needed to promote ankle dorsiflexion.

Swing

During swing, the pelvis rotates anterior as the leg moves forward over the treadmill belt while avoiding forward and side-to-side movement of the trunk. If needed, the trainer assists the client in moving the knee through a normal arc by moving the upper hand (on the medial hamstring) backward. The trainer should avoid rapidly and forcefully lifting the knee or pulling the ankle during swing (he or she should not grasp the ankle). The trainer should avoid pulling the leg outward toward the trainer. It is acceptable for the client to adduct slightly during swing so that foot placement is near midline, but not at or crossing the midline. The rate of swing should be the same for both legs. The trainer should wait for heel contact of other trainer before initiating toe-off. The trainer should allow the client to produce as much of the movement as possible, providing the minimal assistance needed to achieve the appropriate pattern.

Swing-to-Stance Transition

During the swing-to-stance transition, the client's weight shifts onto the swing leg AFTER initial contact of the forward foot. The foot contacts the treadmill before lift-off of the other foot, avoiding placement too far forward or ahead of the hip. Foot placement should optimize both stride length and stance width. Proper stance width should be neither too wide nor too narrow. The foot should be positioned at initial contact so that the hip moves directly over the foot at mid-stance, and both legs should reach the same relative anterior position on the treadmill. The level of neuromuscular activity generated should be considered when selecting the placement of the foot. In early stages of retraining these parameters may not appear to have the precise kinematics, but a particular stride position for each client will result in the best neural pattern.

The trainer's hand placements when assisting are critical to facilitating the appropriate neural pattern for stepping. To assist the client in achieving stance, the trainer should rotate the upper hand to the anterior, proximal tibia at the patellar tendon and simultaneously place the lower hand on the heel to produce a counter-force to assist knee extension and foot placement. Knee extension should be achieved at initial foot contact, rather than trying to establish extension later during stance. Foot placement can vary from the heel to the entire foot making contact with the treadmill. A heel–toe pattern at heel strike is not expected in early training but will be a goal in the later stages of recovery.

Body Weight Support on the Treadmill Operator

To optimize the session time on the treadmill, maximize load-bearing, and provide smooth, consistent therapy, the trainer operating the BWST must take an active role in the therapy session. The operator provides instructions for maintaining good alignment, positioning, and stepping by carefully watching the session and giving verbal cues to the client, hip trainer, and leg trainers. The operator adjusts the BWS and the treadmill speed to maintain optimal stepping and achieve the specific goals of each training session.

Step Adaptability

The aim of step adaptability training is to focus on allowing the neuromuscular system to independently achieve postural control and stepping. Independence from manual facilitation is the first objective while maintaining postural control and coordinated stepping. The focus initially is independence at the trunk (hips and legs may be assisted), then the trunk and pelvis (legs may be assisted, Fig. 5-2a), and finally independence at the trunk,

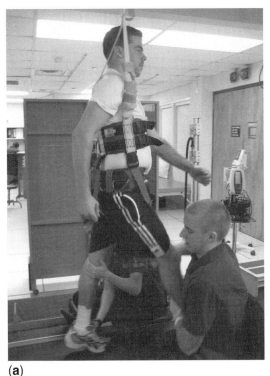 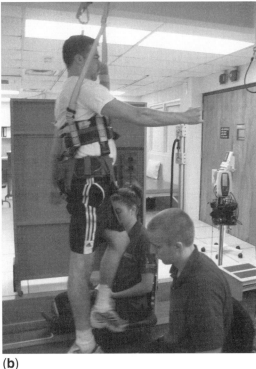

(a)   (b)

FIG 5-2 a, b. Step adaptability.

hips, and legs (Fig. 5-2b). The treadmill speed and BWS are altered to allow independence from the assistance of the trainers at the designated body segments.

Step adaptability proceeds from the treadmill speed and BWS used in the last bout of step retraining and usually requires slowing the treadmill speed and raising the BWS. While stepping, the treadmill speed is gradually decreased until independence in trunk, pelvis, and leg control is achieved. If independence is not achieved before reaching a speed of 0.6 mph, the BWS is then increased until independence is achieved or until the heels begin to rise from the treadmill belt. The usual kinematics of stepping may be compromised during step adaptability but is allowed in order to focus on independence. As independence progresses, the BWS is lowered first before increasing the treadmill speed to afford the translation to overground earlier, since only treadmill speed can be altered overground and an important principle involves avoiding weight-bearing on the arms.

Stand Retraining

Stand training is needed for clients who cannot stand independently overground because of the inability to control the trunk and pelvis. Stand training bouts are interspersed into the step training sessions to improve postural control and balance. During stand training

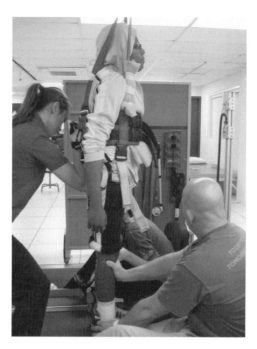

FIG 5-3 Stand retraining.

assistance by the BWS, manual facilitation, hand placement, and verbal cues are used to provide the necessary sensory cues for generating upright postural control (Fig. 5-3). The client's posture should be upright with the head aligned over the shoulders, the shoulders over the trunk, and the upper body in line with the pelvis and the legs (knees, ankles, and feet). The head and trunk should remain in this upright and extended (neutral) position. The pelvis should avoid tilting in the anterior, posterior, or lateral directions while maintaining full, active knee extension.

The BWS should be set as low as possible during stand retraining, allowing the trainers to assist the client in maintaining full, active knee extension and in maintaining good pelvic positioning and full trunk extension with good kinematics. If the client loses the ideal standing position (i.e., flexion at the trunk), the trainers should instruct the client to bring herself or himself back up, as the trainers provide only enough manual and BWS assistance as necessary to regain good posture. Verbal cues are used to help the client maintain an ideal standing position.

Stand Adaptability

The aim of stand adaptability training is to focus on allowing the neuromuscular system to independently achieve upright posture during weight-bearing with independence from BWS and from manual assistance of the trainers. Independence from manual facilitation is the first objective while maintaining postural control and balance during standing.

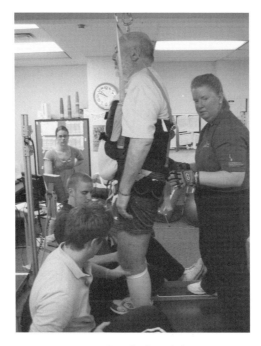

FIG 5-4 Stand adaptability.

The focus initially is independence at the trunk (hips and legs may be assisted, Fig. 5-4), then the trunk and pelvis (legs may be assisted), and finally independence at the trunk, hips, and legs. The BWS can be lowered while the client maintains good trunk, pelvic, and leg kinematics and posture until full body weight load is achieved without manual assistance. Skill in stand adaptability advances as the client incorporates arm use while standing (i.e., reach, lift, grasp, transport, hold), performs transitions in standing (sit to stand), and maintains standing balance if perturbed.

Team Roles

Client

The client is responsible for attending and participating in each session. The frequency of sessions begins five times per week and in the later stages of recovery can be gradually reduced to three times per week, although if possible 5 days per week should be retained. The client assists in goal setting by identifying individual goals and needs and reassesses achievements with the physical therapist/lead trainer and trainer team. Factors that limit achievement of independent walking on the treadmill and independent walking overground are identified and reassessed. The client reports any change in comfort or ability during the actual training session or at home. Practice and decision making beyond the clinic in the home and community by the client consistent with the Locomotor Training guidelines can advance recovery of the neuromuscular system. An active partnership between the client and the trainers in the training process, goal setting, and decision making is encouraged.

Team Leader

The team leader is responsible for implementing the intervention according to the principles and progression guidelines with the team of trainers. The leader is the primary contact for communication with the client concerning the intervention, goals, instructions, and progression. The goals for each session are discussed with the client and the team. Factors that limit achievement of independent walking are identified on the treadmill and overground, directing goal setting and community integration activities. The team leader, in conjunction with the team, sets and alters training parameters and goals, including BWS, treadmill speed, and manual assistance. The team leader may provide manual facilitation at any trainer position on the treadmill and directs the overground and community integration components of the session. Verbal communication within the team is necessary during the training session. The client's physiological response to the training is monitored by every team member; however, the lead trainer may decide whether a session should be terminated or suspended to monitor vital signs or check skin or otherwise. The lead trainer completes the daily documentation recording the session and identifies the next day's training goals. A daily log sheet can facilitate goal setting and prioritization.

Table 5-1 outlines each trainer's roles during stepping.

Hip Trainer

The hip trainer communicates directly with the client. He or she stands just behind the client on the treadmill and therefore can easily monitor the client for signs of fatigue, discomfort, or inadequate stepping consistency and pattern that may require stopping or pausing. The trainer can readily provide encouragement and instructional cues to the client. Such verbal cues are sought first, then manual facilitation, for head position, trunk control, weight transfer, and pelvic motion. Feedback is provided to the team leader concerning the client's response to training. The hip trainer must coordinate training with the leg trainers and be responsive to changes in the stepping pattern.

Leg Trainers

The leg trainers communicate with the client concerning instructions for leg movements or positions (e.g., step length, step back, step width). The leg trainers communicate with one another and the hip trainer to coordinate stepping with pelvic/trunk motion. They provide feedback to the lead trainer concerning training parameters and client response to the training. The leg trainers respond to changes in the BWS and treadmill.

Any trainer and/or the client can request that the training stop or pause for any reason, such as fatigue compromising performance, discomfort or pain, compromised safety, or a pattern of walking that is not consistent with the goal. Communication needs to occur and would be best while training is paused or stopped.

TABLE 5-1 Coordinating Trainer Roles During Stepping

Leg trainer 1*	Leg trainer 2*	Hip trainer	BWST operator
(stance phase)	*(swing phase)*	*(both phases)*	*(both phases)*
Extension of hip and knee	Flexion of hip and knee	Maintain upright trunk and rotate hip back (leg 1) and forward (leg 2) along longitudinal axis.	Cue client, leg trainers, and hip trainer. Adjust the BWS and speed.
Upper hand Place web of hand at patellar tendon. Provide just enough force to achieve knee extension, avoiding hyperextension. Lower hand Place web of hand at tibialis anterior (T.A.), stabilizing dorsum of foot if client tends to evert or invert.	Upper hand Move own arm backwards through mid-swing. Guide knee through swing via a pull at the medial hamstring tendon. Rotate hand back to the patellar tendon at terminal swing. Lower hand Avoid grasping the ankle during mid-swing.	Pull back on rear handle of harness vest, if needed, to assist with upright trunk. Pull back (leg 1) and forward (leg 2) on lateral handle of pelvic band by shifting and rotating own body while keeping arms rigid. Prevent backward, forward, and side-to-side movement of trunk.	Provide feedback on the coordination between the two leg trainers (equal stride length, etc.). Provide feedback on stepping cadence (i.e., going faster or slower than the treadmill or opposite leg). Provide feedback on trunk alignment. Provide feedback on hip rotation and position.

(continued)

TABLE 5-1 *(Continued)*

Leg trainer 1*	Leg trainer 2*	Hip trainer	BWST operator
(stance to swing)	*(swing to stance)*	*(both phases)*	*(both phases)*
Transition from extension to flexion of hip and knee	transition from flexion to extension of hip and knee	maintain upright trunk, rotate hip forward (leg 1) and backward (leg 2) and shift weight to leg 2.	Cue client, leg trainers and hip trainer. Adjust the BWS and speed
Upper hand	Upper hand	Pull back on rear handle of harness vest if needed, to assist with upright trunk.	Provide feedback on timing of weight shift.
Rotate hand from the patellar tendon to the medial hamstring tendon (medially and upwardly).	Finish rotating hand to front of the knee.	Push forward (leg 1) and backward (leg 2) on lateral handle of pelvic band by shifting and rotating own body while keeping arms rigid.	Provide feedback to leg trainers on transition speed.
Press on tendon with the top two fingers.	Provide just enough force to the patellar tendon so that the knee is extended at initial contact.		Check for double-limb support.
Lower hand	Avoid pushing on the patella.	Prevent backward, forward, and side-to-side movement of trunk.	Provide feedback to the trainers.
Assist foot clearance at lift-off by gently pushing upward at the T.A. of the ankle.	Lower hand		
Keep fingers open and avoid grasping the Achilles tendon.	Rotate the fingers to the Achilles tendon at the end of swing and assist the foot through to initial contact.		

*Reverse leg trainer directions as transition to second phase of step cycle

Body Weight Support and Treadmill Operator

This position is integral to a successful step training session. The BWST operator is an experienced trainer and must be attuned to the goals of the session and to the client's response to the training parameters. The operator has a distinct view of the training response and thus can provide changes to the training parameters or directions to the trainers and feedback to the lead trainer to improve the training session and client response.

6

Introduction to Overground Assessment and Community Integration

Chapter Outline

Chapter Objectives

The objectives of Chapter 6 are to:

1. Describe the role and goals of assessment overground in Locomotor Training.
2. Describe the role and goals of community integration in Locomotor Training.

3. Describe overground assessment in Locomotor Training applied to the tasks of trunk stability, sit to stand, standing, and walking.
4. Describe community integration in Locomotor Training applied to the tasks of trunk stability, sit to stand, standing, and walking.
5. Discuss considerations when introducing assistive devices in community integration.

Summary

The overground assessment and community integration components of Locomotor Training combined with the step training component capitalize on the continually changing capacity of the nervous system driven by the retraining. Physical therapists and trainers must be skillful while applying the Locomotor Training principles as they translate this capacity to overground environments. The team will implement clinical decisions to progress the client and balance compensation needed for daily life without compromising recovery. These decisions will determine the rate and success of the recovery of mobility, postural control, standing, and walking for their clients.

Assessment overground allows the client and trainer to assess the client's comfort and capacity to maintain postural control and walk in the overground environment. Community integration prepares the client for functioning at home and in the community. The client and therapist face new challenges in these environments where body weight support (BWS) and manual facilitation are absent. The therapist's role is to limit compensation and continuously encourage recovery and independence while providing succinct and immediate verbal cues. The primary goal of both overground assessment and community integration is to translate the capacity of the nervous system developed during step training to walking at home and in the community. The Locomotor Training principles are applied in these two training environments consistently as during step training.

Trainer facilitation must be minimized during overground assessment and eliminated for community integration. Bracing is not used during overground assessment and the least restrictive assistive device is selected for use in community integration, along with instructions for how to use the device that are consistent with the Locomotor Training principles. Devices are preferred that encourage an upright, symmetrical trunk posture; limit loading on the arms; promote maximal loading on the legs; allow reciprocal arm swing; maintain normal walking speeds; and allow preservation of a reciprocal gait pattern with hip, knee, and ankle flexion and extension. Limitations to independent walking are identified during assessment overground and community integration and are specifically targeted in the next step training session. Such limitations are addressed more effectively during step training on the treadmill since body weight load, treadmill speed, and manual facilitation are easily adjusted so the client can achieve optimal stepping and retraining of the neuromuscular system in a safe environment. The therapist also instructs the client in activities and strategies to advance functional recovery in the home and community. The Locomotor Training principles are thus applied during training on the treadmill, walking overground, and daily activities within the home and community. The following sections provide guidelines for translating the Locomotor Training principles from the step training environment to the overground and community environments.

Overground assessment provides the client the opportunity to independently attempt perform tasks needed to return to daily activities including sitting, trunk stability, transitioning from supine to sit and sit to stand, standing, and walking using the capacity of the retrained nervous system. Assessment overground occurs in each session (also see Chapters 7 and 8, phasing and progression) and immediately follows step training on the treadmill. The change from step training on the treadmill with BWS to overground results in the loss of (1) speed and momentum driven by the treadmill; (2) BWS assist; (3) upright posture and balance assist; and (4) optimal facilitation of leg, pelvis, and trunk movements. The trainer and client identify any limitations to achieving these motor tasks so they can be targeted in the next step training session. For example, if the client has difficulty with independent trunk control during weight shift overground, improving this ability will be a goal of the next step training adaptability session. Other areas of concern that may need to be addressed in step training include balance, upright posture, speed, body weight load on legs, weight shift, and proper kinematics. The primary goals are addressed during stand and step adaptability (goal setting and progression will be addressed in detail in Chapters 7 and 8).

Trunk Stability

The client's goal is to be able to maintain the head and trunk upright over the pelvis during sitting, standing, and walking and to maintain posture when transitioning between body positions. Trunk stability is the most important prerequisite for progressing to independent sitting, standing, and stepping as well as for transfers, mobility, and wheelchair propulsion. The trainer assesses the client's stability, balance, and posture in many areas including transitions from supine to sitting, during sitting (Fig. 6-1), and in maneuvers of trunk extension, as well as during standing and walking. Throughout all of these tasks, the client should focus on maintaining good posture and alignment with the head up, shoulders back and even, and the abdominal muscles tightened. The trainer corrects posture and alignment as necessary by giving verbal cues.

Sit to Stand

Assessment of the client's capacity to independently perform sit to stand begins with the client seated at the edge of a mat with feet flat on the ground. The trainer should instruct the client to avoid using arm support. First, the ability to initiate weight-bearing on the legs without using arms is assessed. If the client is unable to shift the weight, then goals for step training and community integration are set to improve acceptance of weight-bearing on the legs. Next, the ability to raise the body off the mat is assessed; if this is achieved without fully standing upright, then dynamic weight shift is targeted as a primary goal. Next, transitioning to sit to stand with appropriate trunk posture is assessed. Trainer facilitation is allowed only on the pelvis and legs. This is intended to focus recovery on the trunk stability first. Once independence is achieved at the trunk, then the focus of recovery progresses to the pelvis and finally to the legs. When the trunk is independent, the pelvis is now assessed, but independence must occur with both trunk and pelvis unassisted.

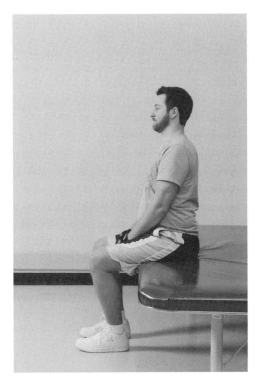

FIG 6-1 Overground assessment: trunk posture in sitting.

The legs may be assisted in this step. Finally, all body segments are evaluated during the sit-to-stand transition without manual facilitation. Throughout the client's progression toward recovery of the ability to transition from sit to stand, the current limitation is addressed as a primary goal during step training and community integration.

Stand

In overground assessment of standing, the focus should be on standing posture beginning with the trunk and then the pelvis prior to the independence of the legs. Proper posture is a prerequisite to standing and walking without BWS. The client must develop comfort in safely standing independently with dynamic balance and endurance. Standing is a dynamic task; knees should not "lock" or hyperextend. The trainer should accurately and continuously provide verbal cues to the client. The first stage of assessment should be in assessing the client's ability to maintain the trunk upright without manual facilitation of the trunk (facilitation may be provided if needed to the pelvis and legs; Fig. 6-2). Then the ability to maintain upright posture with both trunk and pelvis independent from manual facilitation is assessed. Next complete independence during standing with sufficient endurance is evaluated. Finally, dynamic balance while leaning and reaching should be achieved (Fig. 6-3a and 6-3b). Throughout the client's progression toward recovery of standing, the current limitation is addressed as a primary goal during step training and community integration.

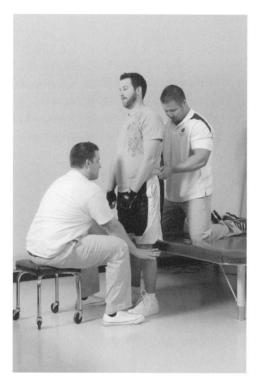

FIG 6-2 Overground assessment: standing.

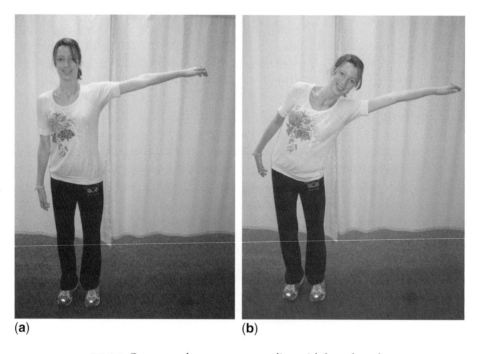

(a)   (b)

FIG 6-3 Overground assessment: standing with lateral reach.

Initiating Walking

In overground assessment of walking, the focus should be on upright posture while achieving a stride position, shifting weight, rotating the pelvis, and moving the legs in an appropriate extension and flexion pattern to propel the body forward to achieve repetitive steps.

The trainers evaluate the aspects of initiating stepping—upright alignment, stride position, or weight shift—that will then be goals for the next step training session. Trainers should start the client in a standing position (upright posture), and first assess the ability to shift weight laterally as well as back and forth in the stride position (Fig. 6-4a and 6-4b). Next the ability to independently achieve the stride position is assessed, followed by appropriate kinematics during flexion and extension of the legs while walking. The client's head and trunk should be extended and the shoulders externally rotated. Trainers will continuously assess that the overall body kinematics are appropriate for an upright posture while walking overground. Throughout the client's progression toward recovery of walking, the current limitation is addressed as a primary goal during step training and community integration.

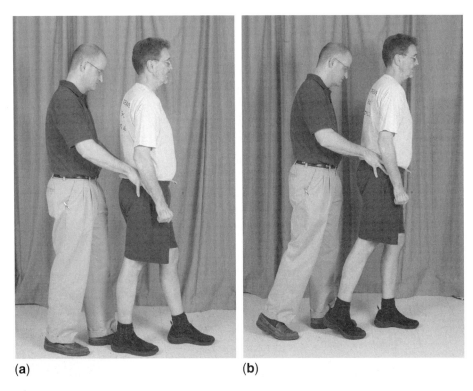

(a)　　　　**(b)**

FIG 6-4 Overground assessment. **a.** Initiating walking: upright posture in stride position. **b.** Initiating walking: weight shift.

Community integration prepares the client for functioning in the home and community and translates the capacity of the retrained neuromuscular system into its use in everyday tasks and activities. During the therapy session, community integration occurs immediately following overground assessment. Community integration addresses the development of independence for mobility, sitting, transferring, transitioning from sit to stand, standing, and walking in the home and community while limiting compensation and encouraging recovery. The emphasis is on maximizing opportunities to incorporate the Locomotor Training principles into everyday activities and tasks. For example, the trainers should encourage such activities as standing while brushing teeth or preparing meals and limiting the use of arms for weight-bearing. The client is encouraged to incorporate the legs into daily tasks, especially for load-bearing. If asymmetries exist between the legs, use of the more involved leg is emphasized. Several practice repetitions performed in the clinic ensure that the client understands and can perform the movements independently at home or with the assistance of a caregiver, family member, or friend.

The client should always be encouraged and allowed to attempt the movement before assistance is provided. Even though the client may be unable to perform the task, allowing him or her to first attempt the required movement contributes to more effective relearning. If the client attempts the movement using a compensation strategy (e.g., throwing the trunk forward or backward) or the speed of the movement is slow, trainers provide verbal cues to correct the movement, and then facilitate if needed. Trainers provide and gauge manual facilitation to achieve proper kinematics of the movement and maximal independence by the client. Trainers should always limit their assistance and continuously encourage independent attempts at movements by the client.

If the client is ambulatory, the therapist promotes an ambulation strategy based on the Locomotor Training principles. Immediate goals are addressed that are consistent with those identified during step training adaptability and evaluated during assessment overground. The therapist instructs the client in use of the least restrictive assistive device that provides the needed safety and maximum independence and is most consistent with the Locomotor Training principles. Multiple goals for ambulation, such as speed, load, independence, and endurance, may be addressed during home and community ambulation by using different assistive devices. The physical therapist assesses the client's limits to achieving independent and safe community ambulation during overground assessment and then instructs him or her in home activities during community integration.

Functional Goals for Mobility

A client's ability to transition from lying to sitting, maintain sitting, transfer from bed to wheelchair and onto other surfaces, propel a manual wheelchair, and maintain stability while riding in a car are all functional goals early in recovery. The recovery of trunk stability is critical to achieving these tasks with the least amount of compensation. Trainers should identify activities for the client to perform at home that will challenge the client's independence and endurance until she or he is able to maintain trunk stability consistently without assistance. Trunk stability can be challenged and developed by assisting the client into good sitting trunk posture and asking the client to hold the position. Trunk activation can be promoted by performing sit-ups, partial sit-ups in targeted ranges requiring concentric or eccentric muscle activity, and reverse sit-ups by extending the trunk from a forward-flexed position, and applying resistance to trunk flexion and then extension in sitting. As the client recovers and can maintain the trunk independently and indefinitely, then the trainers should challenge the posture with balance tasks requiring trunk movement outside of the base of support or greater demand to maintain a static trunk posture (e.g., reaching, lifting, and allowing the trunk to flex forward or extend backward). During community integration in the clinic, the therapist/ trainer demonstrates these techniques, and then these exercises can be performed in the home and community to increase the amount of practice and repetition and accelerate recovery.

If the wheelchair is currently used for overground mobility, the Locomotor Training principles should be integrated and opportunities to continue to challenge the neuromuscular system should be identified and implemented. The client is instructed to avoid using the back support whenever possible to challenge trunk strength and stability. When transferring, load-bearing through the legs should be emphasized by removing the footrests, positioning the feet under the client and on the ground. The weight shift is then onto the legs (and arms, as needed), but a shared load with increasing load-bearing by the legs versus the arms (Fig. 6-5a). Activation of the trunk into extension during the transfer also is reinforced (Fig. 6-5b and 6-5c). These activities will promote neuromuscular activity for eventually achieving sit to stand. If the client is using a power wheelchair, then the team should also include activities to strengthen the arms, such as pushing up the body off the chair. When possible, the team should have the client begin pushing a manual

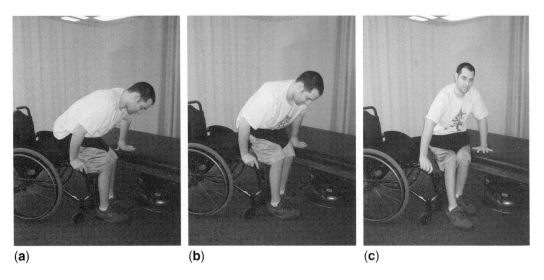

(a) (b) (c)

FIG 6-5 Community integration. **a–c**. Client transferring with emphasis on load-bearing through the legs, trunk extension, and decreased load-bearing by the arms.

chair for periods throughout the day. In community integration, trunk posture and control are emphasized throughout the experiences of daily living, from dressing to brushing one's teeth to getting in and out of bed. Throughout all activities of daily life, using the neuromuscular system below the lesion or using the affected body segment to achieve a functional goal should be prioritized, while also reducing compensation whenever possible.

Sit to Stand

A client's ability to independently transition from sit to stand is required for activities of daily life such as getting out of bed or in and out of a car, efficient toileting, and accessing community venues, including school, work, theaters, and so forth. Recovering the ability to transition from sit to stand can be more difficult than standing and should be targeted for progression early in recovery. Initiating weight-bearing on the legs whenever possible will accelerate achieving this functional goal. The therapist/trainers should instruct the client to complete exercises such as repetitive partial weight-bearing on the legs from sitting and exercises to strengthen the muscles needed for knee and hip extension. The client should take advantage of any opportunity to bear weight and attempt extension using transfers throughout the day to partially load the legs and activate extensor muscles even when the transfer is assisted. As the client's ability recovers, an assistive device such as a walker can be incorporated for practice of initiating weight-bearing and rising to stand while at home (Fig. 6-6a and 6-6b). The kinematics specific to the task of coming to stand are reinforced even with a device or support while in the home and community.

Caregivers, family members, and friends can be instructed on how to safely facilitate manually at the trunk and/or legs for practice outside the therapy session. As soon as possible the loading on the arms should be minimal and used only for assisting with balance. Independence from manual facilitation, from an assistive device, or from use of the arms to move from sitting to standing is an important goal for community integration. If such support is necessary to achieve independence at home, training continues during step training in the clinic to increase the neuromuscular capacity to eventually achieve complete independence.

Stand

A client's ability to stand is important not only for reaching many functional goals, but also for improving overall health by increasing cardiovascular and respiratory function, bone density, and muscle mass. The initial focus for standing during community integration is to instruct and prepare the client to be able to stand safely in the home. Proper trunk control, alignment, and posture and load-bearing through the legs are emphasized. Use of a full-length mirror can facilitate the process, as the client can observe his or her own posture and make the needed adjustments. If the arms are needed to assist balance, then minimizing the load-bearing through the arms is encouraged. The client may initially require assistance for balance, and using horizontal poles allows the trainer to set the height to minimize weight-bearing with the arms (Fig. 6-7). The horizontal poles are used for balance assist but not for upper extremity load-bearing, as often occurs with standard assistive devices. The trainer should continuously assess the degree of support

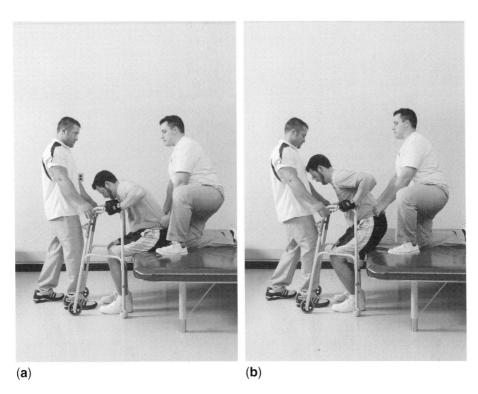

(a)   (b)

FIG 6-6 Community integration **a, b.** Sit-to-stand practice in preparation for home and community. Kinematics specific to the task are practiced even with an assistive device to promote weight-bearing and activation of leg and trunk muscles.

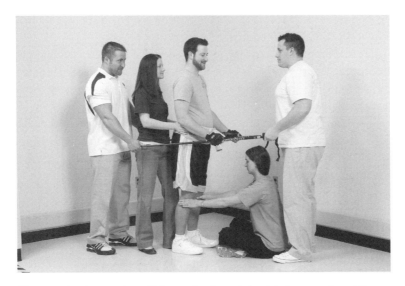

FIG 6-7 Community integration. Using poles for minimal balance assist while promoting standing and load-bearing through legs overground.

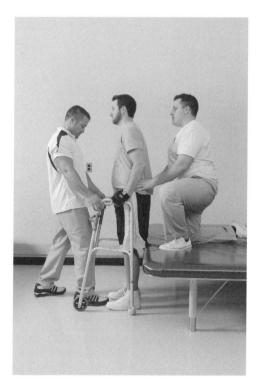

FIG 6-8 Community integration. Use of a walker as practice for standing in the home and community.

that is necessary, as the goal is to maximize weight-bearing on the legs and to minimize arm support. To promote successful standing with trunk alignment, the client should develop an awareness of even distribution of weight on the legs by frequently shifting weight between the two limbs.

In the home, a client may require assistance into the standing position. Early in recovery, an assistive device may be introduced and manual facilitation may be needed at the trunk, pelvis, and/or knees (Fig. 6-8). If facilitation is necessary, then using intermittent rather than constant facilitation is preferred to promote activation of the neuromuscular system. Independence from manual facilitation at the trunk should be the first goal. For instance, a walker may be used to provide some trunk support and balance with minimal upper extremity load-bearing, with manual facilitation provided at the pelvis and knees to achieve standing. The next goal is independence at the pelvis, followed by the knees, and ultimately without use of the assistive device.

The ability to balance can be progressed by providing additional challenges to the client such as raising an arm, reaching, or moving the body outside the base of support.

As the ability to stand recovers, the skill can be incorporated into daily activities such as brushing teeth, grooming, preparing meals, and washing dishes. Any time that the client can load-bear and stand during a meaningful, functional task at home or in the community, then the client should take advantage of the opportunity to promote recovery. Endurance should also be progressed by increasing the number of times an individual stands throughout the day and the length of time continuously standing.

Walking

Walking is a primary goal for individuals with neurologic injury and disease and when recovered improves quality of life by giving full access to the home and community. There are many challenges to achieving a good walking pattern overground. They include maintaining an upright posture and balance while walking, controlling the speed of walking, supporting the body with full leg weight-bearing, moving and placing the legs with proper kinematics and timing, and developing independence and confidence. The goal during walking is to continue the pattern of "stance, transition, swing, transition" with an emphasis on upright posture, stride position, and weight shift.

The first goal overground during the recovery of walking is to be able to initiate weight shift from the stride position. From the stride position, the client rapidly shifts weight forward onto the front leg and unloads the extended back leg to initiate stepping overground. This movement is critical for providing the correct sensory cues to the nervous system. The client is asked to shift weight to one leg, flex the hip and knee of the other leg slightly to lift, move the leg backward by extending the hip and knee, and then place the foot on the ground and shift weight onto the back leg. Trainers will encourage and assist the client using cue words, but should assist the client only if necessary. Hip extension and the timing of unloading with initiation of swing should be emphasized to take advantage of the intrinsic capacity of the spinal cord circuits to initiate swing initially and throughout sequential steps. Use of parallel, handheld horizontal poles on each side of the client may promote greater walking speed and provide stability with minimal weight-bearing on the arms while walking overground. An alternative is for a trainer (or two) to hold the client's hand and promote arm swing while walking (Fig. 6-9). It is advantageous to immediately transition from step retraining (treadmill) to walking overground to take advantage of the enhanced physiological state of the nervous system for walking.

Good stepping during community integration is promoted using the same strategies used in step training on the treadmill and overground walking training. For example, the client is encouraged to initiate stepping using exactly the same procedure (upright posture, stride position, and weight shift), even though the assistive device may be used. Walking at faster speeds may promote a good stepping pattern. Advanced ambulation activities may be introduced in this component as well. The goal is for clients to be able to successfully negotiate their environment, to react to a changing environment, and to meet their own behavioral goals for community ambulation. Examples of advanced activities are walking at variable speeds, starting and stopping at different speeds, turning around and navigating corners, climbing stairs, and negotiating obstacles. Trips or stumbles occasionally occur during everyday walking. If the client stumbles during community integration, encourage him or her to regain balance by using the legs rather than using the arms. Specific goals may be identified based on the individual's home and community environment.

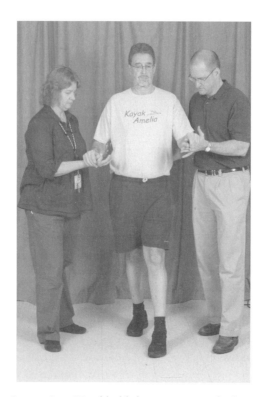

FIG 6-9 Community integration. Hand holds by two trainers facilitating arm swing can be used to increase the client's walking speed and minimize upper extremity load-bearing.

Introducing Assistive Devices

In making the transition to home and community, an assistive device may be introduced to achieve endurance, safety, and independence. It is critical to select the "least restrictive device"—that is, the one most consistent with the Locomotor Training principles. Devices are preferred that encourage an upright, symmetrical trunk posture; limit loading on the arms; promote maximal loading on the legs; allow reciprocal arm swing; maintain normal walking speeds; and allow preservation of a reciprocal gait pattern with hip, knee, and ankle flexion and extension.

Consideration of the Locomotor Training principles should be made when selecting a device in order to achieve safe and independent community ambulation. The selection of particular devices depends on the current goals. For example, a wheeled walker may be used to achieve a goal of independent ambulation in the community at a certain speed of walking and endurance (Fig. 6-10). Two canes may be more challenging to the trunk and allow coordination of arm and leg movement, but most likely will result in a slower speed of walking by the client in the home (Fig. 6-11). Thus, two devices may be recommended at the same time for use in the home and community. Alternating between the two

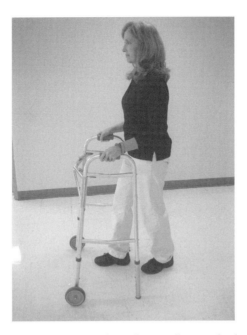

FIG 6-10 Community integration. Use of a rolling walker in the home and community promotes walking at faster speeds, endurance, and independence, though with potential change in kinematics (e.g., loss of upright trunk, hip extension) and greater load-bearing on the arms.

devices provides a continual challenge to the neuromuscular system to improve independence, endurance, or speed, as well as stepping and postural control. As recovery continues, then alternative devices may be introduced to advance skill progression and challenge the nervous system.

A standard assistive device may be modified to be more consistent with the Locomotor Training principles. For example, raising the handle height of a device can minimize weight-bearing on the arms, reinforce loading on the legs, and promote a more upright posture. The client should be instructed to promote the Locomotor Training principles while using an assistive device. For example, the client is instructed to place the foot on the ground before the assistive device (specifically when walking with crutches or canes). This practice encourages weight-bearing and balance control using the legs rather than the arms. While the choice of using one cane instead of two is often viewed as a step towards independence, the use of a single cane or crutch often results in an asymmetrical walking pattern. The client is encouraged to use two single-point canes to facilitate a more symmetrical walking pattern and then if possible progress to none or to one only for uneven terrain or unpredictable circumstances in the community environment. Walking poles offer an alternative to the use of canes and allow a more upright posture and limited weight-bearing on the arms (Fig. 6-12). The poles can also provide minimal stability, again for uneven terrain or unexpected conditions.

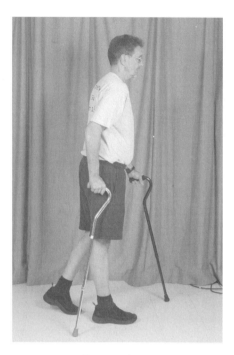

FIG 6-11 Community integration. Walking with two canes permits an upright posture, a kinematic pattern consistent with walking, and reduced upper extremity loading, and greater load-bearing occurs on the legs. Bilateral canes promote a more symmetrical walking pattern as compared to a single cane.

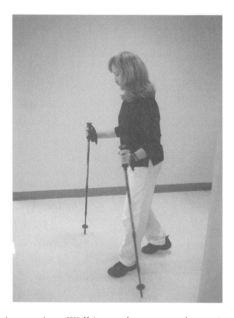

FIG 6-12 Community integration. Walking poles are an alternative to canes and provide upright posture with minimal upper extremity load-bearing.

The components of Locomotor Training, step retraining, overground assessment, and community integration should be synergistic and focus on the same specific goals to progress toward the next phase of recovery. The success of the Locomotor Training intervention depends not only on the quality of the step and stand retraining but also on the intensity of the intervention and the ongoing decisions made by the therapy team and the client. It is essential for clients to incorporate the Locomotor Training principles into their daily life and to continue their progression to recovery in the home and community in addition to the daily therapy session. The final two chapters discuss the guidelines of progression through specific phases of recovery.

7

Phases of Recovery

Chapter Outline

b. Hip Trainer
c. Leg Trainers
d. Assessment
iii. Scoring
D. Step Adaptability
  i. Optimal Client Position
  ii. Trainer Instructions
    a. BWST Operator
    b. Hip Trainer
    c. Leg Trainers
    d. Assessment
  iii. Scoring
III. Abilities During Overground Assessment
A. Sit
  i. Optimal Client Position
  ii. Trainer Instructions
  iii. Scoring
B. Reverse Sit-Up
  i. Optimal Client Position
  ii. Trainer Instructions
  iii. Scoring
C. Sit-Up
  i. Optimal Client Position
  ii. Trainer Instructions
  iii. Scoring
D. Trunk Extension in Sitting
  i. Optimal Client Position
  ii. Trainer Instructions
  iii. Scoring
E. Sit to Stand
  i. Optimal Client Position
  ii. Trainer Instructions
  iii. Scoring
F. Stand
  i. Optimal Client Position
  ii. Trainer Instructions
  iii. Scoring
G. Walking
  i. Optimal Client Position
  ii. Trainer Instructions
  iii. Scoring
IV. Overview of Utilization of Phases of Recovery for Progression
V. Appendix A
A. Phase Scoring Sheet
VI. Appendix B
A. Phase Sheet Cards

Chapter Objectives

The objectives of Chapter 7 are to:

1. Define the four phases of recovery.
2. Understand the definitions of the subphases.
3. Identify training goals for specific phases of recovery.

Summary

The Locomotor Training intervention is implemented by identifying specific goals based on the current phase of recovery. Properly and continuously challenging clients to achieve higher levels of performance is critical to recovery. Therapists and activity-based technicians use the phases of recovery to evaluate the client's current ability and identify training goals and progression strategies to optimize recovery. Even though the accomplished neural plasticity may not have yet resulted in reaching functional goals such as transferring, standing, or improvements in walking, the assessments in the phasing will show more incremental changes in neural recovery. This then gives an indication that the therapy is having a positive effect and should continue. The sequence of implementing these specific goals is based both on the scientific evidence and the experience of many physical therapists who have provided the intervention in research and clinical environments over the past decade.

Introduction to Four Phases of Recovery

There are four general phases of recovery, defined by client ability assessed within two components of Locomotor Training: step training (retraining and adaptability) and overground assessment (adaptability). Full recovery is defined as the neuromuscular system's ability to execute a motor task as prior to injury and no longer needing any form of compensation. The phase of recovery of the motor task will define the ability of the individual to achieve the specific motor task without compensation. This continuum proceeds from unable to complete the task to achieving full recovery by executing the task as done pre-injury. A full phase assessment is recommended after approximately every 20 Locomotor Training sessions to provide specific information related to how a client is responding to the therapy. We recommend that you recheck daily during overground assessment the three "lagging" or lowest-scored factors to guide your daily goals for step retraining and community integration activities.

The body weight support on the treadmill (BWST) affords a permissive environment in which to assess the capacity of the nervous system to stand and generate steps in a safe environment. The capacity of the nervous system is assessed by identifying the treadmill speed, BWS, and level of facilitation needed to generate the optimal stepping pattern. The independence of the nervous system is assessed by identifying the treadmill speed and BWS where independence from manual facilitation occurs. Overground assessment defines the capacity of the neuromuscular system without the benefit of the BWST, assistive devices, or physical assistance.

Phase 1 is the earliest stage of recovery. The individual is severely limited in the overground environment and needs maximal compensation for mobility and ambulation with use of a wheelchair. Often the individual experiences symptoms of multiple secondary conditions related to neurologic injury. The primary focus is retraining posture and increasing endurance.

Phase 2 is the mid-stage of recovery. The individual has regained mobility in the overground environment but needs significant compensation for standing and walking. The primary focus is retraining of the nervous system to stand.

Phase 3 is the later stage of recovery. The individual has regained mobility and the ability to stand but needs significant compensation to ambulate in the home and community. The primary focus is retraining the nervous system to walk.

Phase 4 is the final stage of recovery. The primary focus is on increasing endurance and speed and adapting to the environmental challenges while returning to pre-injury physical activities. Compensation, including physical assistance and assistive devices, is not required.

Abilities During Step Training

The step training environment uses the BWST and manual facilitation to assess the capacity and independence of the nervous system to maintain posture, stand, and generate steps in a safe environment. The capacity of the nervous systems is assessed by identifying the treadmill speed and BWS to generate the optimal standing or stepping pattern with or without manual facilitation (retraining). The independence of the nervous system is assessed by identifying the treadmill speed (stepping) and BWS (stepping and standing) where independence from manual facilitation occurs (adaptability). There are four areas of assessment during step training: (1) stand retraining, (2) stand adaptability, (3) step retraining, and (4) step adaptability. The goal of the step training evaluation is to determine the BWS (and speed when stepping) needed for retraining and independence at various body segments when the client is standing and stepping. Standing and stepping should occur only long enough to obtain this objective. During stand retraining and step retraining the BWS level (and speed when stepping) are assessed as follows:

Hip Trainer: trunk and pelvis
Left Trainer: left knee and ankle
Right Trainer: right knee and ankle
BWST Operator: controls and records the BWS (and treadmill speed) when independence at each body segment is reported by the trainers

Stand Retraining

Optimal Client Position
Upright posture with head, shoulders, and trunk extended, the pelvis properly positioned under the head and shoulders, and the knees extended and ankles positioned at neutral to adequately maintain body weight using manual facilitation when needed.

Trainer Instructions

The goal of stand retraining is to provide the maximum level of loading on the legs with the most appropriate kinematics. Stand retraining reveals the ability of the neuromuscular system to bear weight. The recorded value is BWS. Facilitation may be provided during retraining to achieve the best posture and position (Fig. 7-1).

BWST Operator

The BWST operator starts with the weight at the baseline BWS, then continuously decreases the support until the BWS reaches 0%, or the lowest level at which posture and position of the head, trunk, pelvis, and legs are maintained. The operator should continuously evaluate the client while adjusting the BWS.

Hip Trainer

The hip trainer gives assistance as needed to the pelvis and trunk while BWS is being decreased, maintaining appropriate posture of a standing position.

Leg Trainers

The leg trainers apply sensory cues at the patellar tendon and Achilles tendon, keeping the leg extended. The legs should have a slight bend—just enough so that the legs are neither hyperextended nor locked into extension.

Assessment

BWS should start at 75% of the client's weight or at the BWS at which both of the client's heels are still on the treadmill. This is now considered the client's baseline BWS.

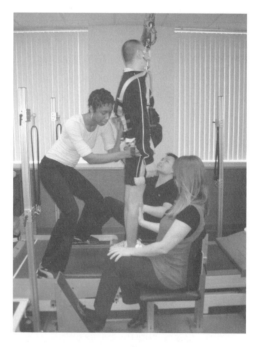

FIG 7-1 Stand retraining.

The BWS starts at the baseline level and is lowered continuously to allow client to bear as much weight as possible through the lower extremities. Facilitation is provided by each trainer (at the trunk, pelvis, knees, and ankles) as needed to achieve maximal weight-bearing. The BWS is lowered to the lowest level at which that the trainer's facilitation is sufficient to maintain the appropriate kinematics and ensure the client's safety for at least 5 minutes. It is not necessary to continue for the 5 minutes to determine the level of BWS, but the load must be considered appropriate for a meaningful training bout. This BWS is recorded and the stand retraining assessment has been completed. The trainer refers to the Phases of Recovery Assessment scoring and marks the appropriate subphase according to the definition given. BWS is recorded in increments of 5% (always rounding to higher value).

Scoring

- Phase 1A. Stand retraining: ≥40% BWS. Client must remain above 40% BWS for trainers to maintain proper posture of head, shoulders, and trunk and positioning of pelvis, legs, and ankles. At BWS of 39% or below, trainers are unable to maintain posture and/or positioning continuously for at least 5 minutes.
- Phase 1B. Stand retraining: 20–39% BWS. Client must remain between 20% and 39% BWS for trainers to maintain proper posture of head, shoulders, and trunk and positioning of pelvis, legs and ankles. At BWS 19% or below, trainers are unable to maintain proper posture and/or positioning continuously for at least 5 minutes.
- Phase 1C–2A: Not applicable
- Phase 2B. Stand retraining: 10–19% BWS. Client must remain between 10% and 19% BWS for trainers to maintain proper posture of head, shoulders, and trunk and positioning of pelvis, knees, and ankles. At BWS 9% or below, trainers are unable to maintain proper posture and/or positioning continuously for at least 5 minutes.
- Phase 2C–3B: Not applicable
- Phase 3C. Stand retraining: <10% BWS. Client must remain between 0% and 9% BWS for trainers to maintain proper posture of head, shoulders, and trunk and positioning of pelvis, legs, and ankles continuously for at least 5 minutes.
- Phase 4. Stand retraining: Not applicable

Stand Adaptability

Optimal Client Position
Upright posture with head, shoulders, and trunk extended, the pelvis properly positioned under the head and shoulders, and the knees extended and ankles positioned at neutral to adequately maintain body weight. Manual facilitation is not used for the body segments evaluated. Manual facilitation may be provided for those body segments that are not being evaluated.

Trainer Instructions
The goal of stand adaptability is to objectively assess independence at the trunk, pelvis and the knee and ankle of each leg during standing. The assessment is independence at a

particular BWS. The recorded value is BWS and independent body segments. BWS is continuously increased until the hip or leg trainers can remove facilitation from a particular body segment while the client maintains proper posture and position.

BWST Operator

Starting at the stand retraining levels, BWS is continuously increased while observing for appropriate posture and position and safety of client. When the assessment is completed the operator records the appropriate BWS values for trunk, hip, and leg independence and the subphase for stand adaptability.

Hip Trainer

When specifically assessing the trunk, the trainer decreases the facilitation at the trunk while BWS is being increased, attempting to find the lowest BWS at which the client can maintain complete independence of the trunk with proper posture. When assessing the pelvis and legs, assistance is not provided for the trunk. When assessing the pelvis, the trainer decreases assistance at the pelvis while BWS is being increased, attempting to find the lowest BWS at which the client can establish complete independence of the trunk and pelvis. When assessing the legs, the trainer must not provide assistance to the trunk or pelvis.

Leg Trainers

When facilitation is needed, the trainers should use proper sensory cueing at the legs to ensure appropriate kinematics. Assistance can be provided continuously when evaluating the trunk and pelvis. When specifically assessing the legs, the trainer decreases assistance while BWS is being increased, attempting to find the lowest BWS at which the client can to establish complete independence. Both legs must be completely independent with maintained posture and position of the pelvis and extension of the hip and knee and neutral position of the ankle.

Assessment

Starting at the level used for scoring during stand retraining, the BWS is increased continuously while removing facilitation at the body segments. If the baseline BWS is attained without independence at the trunk, pelvis, knee, or ankle, that particular body segment will be deemed as not attaining independence, even if independence can be attained at a higher BWS. The assessment of independence follows this order: (1) trunk, (2) pelvis, and (3) legs. The pelvis is not assessed unless the trunk reaches independence below 20%. If the trunk was not independent below 20%, the BWS is recorded and the stand adaptability assessment has been completed. If the trunk body segment was independent below 20% BWS, the pelvis is assessed. The knees and ankles are not assessed unless the trunk and pelvis are independent below 10%. BWS is increased toward 60%, and when the pelvis is independent, that BWS value is recorded. If the pelvis is not independent at 60%, then the stand adaptability assessment is complete. If the BWS is less than 10% and the trunk and pelvis are independent, then the legs are assessed. If the BWS is more than 10%, the stand adaptability assessment has been completed. If the trunk and pelvis body segments attain independence below 10%, the knees and ankles are assessed. BWS is lowered while the trunk, hips, and legs are independent and the lowest BWS at which this occurs is recorded. If both legs are not independent at less than 10%, the stand adaptability assessment is complete.

Referring to the Phases of Recovery Assessment, the appropriate subphase is marked according to the definition given. BWS is recorded in increments of 5% (always rounding to higher value).

Scoring

- Phase 1A. Stand adaptability: >60% BWS, unable to maintain proper posture at head, shoulders, and trunk without manual facilitation. With BWS greater than 60%, the client's head, shoulders, and/or trunk still require manual facilitation to maintain proper posture. Pelvis, knees, and ankles receive manual facilitation as needed.
- Phase 1B. Stand adaptability: 40–59% BWS, maintain proper posture at head, shoulders, and trunk without manual facilitation. With BWS between 40% and 59% BWS, the client's head, shoulders, and trunk do not require manual facilitation from the trainer to maintain proper posture. Pelvis, knees, and ankles receive manual facilitation as needed.
- Phase 1C. Stand adaptability: 20–39% BWS, maintain proper posture at head, shoulders, and trunk without manual facilitation. With BWS between 20% and 39% BWS, the client's head, shoulders, and trunk do not require manual facilitation from the trainer to maintain proper posture. Pelvis, knees, and ankles receive manual facilitation as needed (Fig. 7-2).

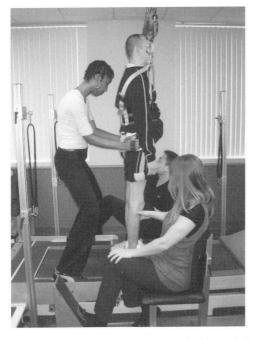

FIG 7-2 Phase 1C: Stand adaptability: BWS 20–39% and able to independently maintain proper posture at trunk.

- Phase 2A. Stand adaptability: <20% BWS, maintain proper posture at head, shoulders, and trunk without manual facilitation. With BWS between 0% and 19%, the client's head, shoulders, and trunk do not require manual facilitation from the trainer to maintain proper posture. Pelvis, knees, and ankles receive manual facilitation as needed.
- Phase 2B. Stand adaptability: 40–59% BWS, maintain proper posture at head, shoulders, and trunk and positioning at pelvis without manual facilitation. With BWS between 40% and 59% BWS, the client's head, shoulders, trunk, and pelvis do not require manual facilitation from the trainer to maintain proper posture and positioning; knees and ankles receive manual facilitation as needed (Fig. 7-3).
- Phase 2C. Stand adaptability: 10–39% BWS, maintain proper posture at head, shoulders, and trunk and positioning at pelvis without manual facilitation. With BWS between 10% and 39%, the client's head, shoulders, trunk, and pelvis do not require manual facilitation from the trainer to maintain proper posture and positioning; knees and ankles receive manual facilitation as needed.
- Phase 3A: Not applicable
- Phase 3B. Stand adaptability: <10% BWS, maintain proper posture at head, shoulders, and trunk and positioning at pelvis. With BWS between 0% and 9%, the client's head, shoulders, trunk, and pelvis do not require manual facilitation from the trainer to maintain proper posture and positioning; knees and ankles receive manual facilitation as needed.

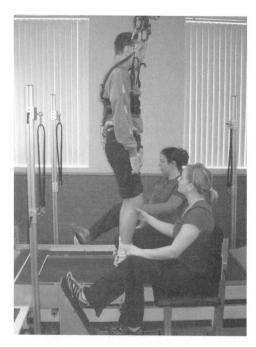

FIG 7-3 Phase 2B: Stand adaptability: BWS 40–59% and independence at trunk and pelvis with proper posture and position.

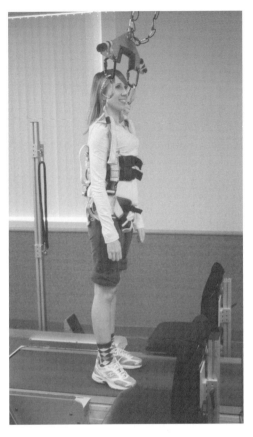

FIG 7-4 Phase 3C: Stand adaptability: BWS <10% used for balance deficits, independence at trunk with proper posture and at pelvis and legs with proper position.

- Phase 3C. Stand adaptability: <10% BWS, maintain proper posture at head, shoulders, and trunk and positioning of pelvis, knees, and ankles. With BWS between 0% and 9%, the client's head, shoulders and trunk, pelvis, knees, and ankles do not require manual facilitation from the trainer to maintain proper posture and positioning. The BWS may be used as a safety for balance deficiencies (Fig. 7-4).
- Phase 4. Stand adaptability: 0% BWS, head, shoulders, trunk posture, and positioning of pelvis, knees, and ankle and ability to balance recovered. With no BWS/harness, the client's head, shoulders, trunk, pelvis, knees, and ankles do not require manual facilitation to maintain proper posture, positioning and balance. The BWS is not used for balance (Fig. 7-5).

Step Retraining

Optimal Client Position
Proper kinematics of the head, shoulders, and trunk; axial alignment of the shoulders, hip, knees, and ankles; pelvis rotation; and kinematics of the hip, knee, and ankles during

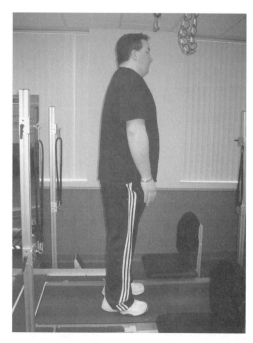

FIG 7-5 Phase 4: Stand adaptability with 0% BWS and able to maintain proper posture at trunk and position of pelvis and legs and balance.

the step cycle should be maintained at pre-injury walking speeds (approximately 2.0–3.4 mph). BWS is adjusted and trainers use manual facilitation to maintain proper kinematics to produce flexion during swing and extension during stance and execute the stance-to-swing and swing-to-stance transitions.

Trainer Instructions

The goal of step retraining is to provide the maximum level of loading on the legs with appropriate kinematics during stepping at pre-injury walking speeds. Step retraining reveals the ability of the neuromuscular system to generate a locomotor pattern when provided with the sensory cues associated with walking. The recorded values are BWS and speed. Manual facilitation may be provided during retraining to achieve the best posture and kinematics while stepping at pre-injury walking speeds.

BWST Operator

Starting at the level of BWS scored for stand adaptability, speed is increased to a normal walking speed (2.0 mph or higher), and then BWS is decreased until trainers begin to lose appropriate kinematics during stepping. BWS is then increased to the level where the best stepping pattern is elicited. Minor adjustments in speed may be required interleaved with changes in BWS while evaluating the client and the stepping pattern.

Hip Trainer

The trainer provides the facilitation at the hips (and trunk if needed) that is required to achieve maximum weight-bearing, proper posture, and appropriate kinematics while stepping.

Leg Trainers

The trainers deliver proper sensory cueing and give facilitation to the knees and ankles that is required to achieve maximum weight-bearing and appropriate kinematics while stepping.

Assessment

Starting with the BWS at the level used for scoring during stand adaptability, treadmill speed is adjusted to attain a normal walking speed. BWS is then continuously decreased to facilitate the best achievable stepping pattern while maintaining appropriate posture and kinematics. Manual facilitation may be provided by each trainer at the trunk, pelvis, knees, and ankles as needed. When the "ideal stepping" pattern is achieved, the BWS is recorded in increments of 5% (always rounding to the higher value) and the treadmill speed is recorded in increments of 0.2 mph.

Scoring

- Phase 1A. Step retraining: >60% BWS. Client must remain above 60% BWS to generate the best stepping pattern with proper kinematics of the head, shoulders, trunk, pelvis, knees, and ankles. At BWS 60% or below, trainers are unable to maintain proper posture and kinematics. Manual facilitation is provided as needed.
- Phase 1B. Step retraining: 55–59% BWS. Client must remain between 55% and 59% BWS to generate the best stepping pattern with proper kinematics of the head, shoulders, trunk, pelvis, knees, and ankles. At BWS 54% or below, trainers are unable to maintain proper posture and kinematics. Manual facilitation is provided as needed (Fig. 7-6).

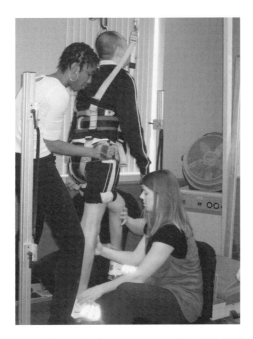

FIG 7-6 Phase 1B: Step retraining, 55–59% BWS.

- Phase 1C. Step retraining: 50–54% BWS. Client must remain between 50% and 54% BWS to generate the best stepping pattern with proper kinematics of the head, shoulders, trunk, pelvis, knees, and ankles. At BWS 49% or below, trainers are unable to maintain proper posture and kinematics. Manual facilitation is provided as needed.
- Phase 2A. Step retraining: 45–49% BWS. Client must remain between 45% and 49% BWS to generate the best stepping pattern with proper kinematics of the head, shoulders, trunk, pelvis, knees, and ankles. At BWS 44% or below, trainers are unable to maintain proper posture and kinematics. Manual facilitation is provided as needed.
- Phase 2B. Step retraining: 40–44% BWS. Client must remain between 40% and 44% BWS to generate the best stepping pattern with proper kinematics of the head, shoulders, trunk, pelvis, knees, and ankles. At BWS 39% or below, trainers are unable to maintain proper posture and kinematics. Manual facilitation is provided as needed (Fig. 7-7).
- Phase 2C. Step retraining: 35–39% BWS. Client must remain between 35% and 39% BWS to generate the best stepping pattern with proper kinematics of the head, shoulders, trunk, pelvis, knees, and ankles. At BWS 34% or below, trainers are unable to maintain proper posture and kinematics. Manual facilitation is provided as needed.
- Phase 3A. Step retraining: 30–34% BWS. Client must remain between 30% and 34% BWS to generate the best stepping pattern with proper kinematics of the head, shoulders, trunk, pelvis, knees, and ankles. At BWS 29% or below, trainers

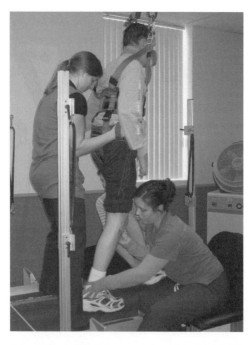

FIG 7-7 Phase 2B: Step retraining, 40–44% BWS.

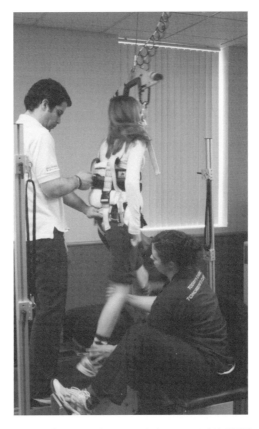

FIG 7-8 Phase 3A: Step retraining, 30–34% BWS.

are unable to maintain proper posture and kinematics. Manual facilitation is provided as needed (Fig. 7-8).

- Phase 3B. Step retraining: 20–29% BWS. Client must remain between 20% and 29% BWS to generate the best stepping pattern with proper kinematics of the head, shoulders, trunk, pelvis, knees, and ankles. At BWS 19% or below, trainers are unable to maintain proper posture and kinematics. Manual facilitation is provided as needed.
- Phase 3C. Step retraining: <20% BWS. Client must remain between 0% and 19% BWS to generate the best stepping pattern and maintain proper posture and kinematics. Manual facilitation is provided as needed.
- Phase 4. Step retraining (running): <50% BWS >3.4 mph. Client must remain between 0% and 49% BWS to generate the best running pattern with proper kinematics. Manual facilitation is provided as needed (Fig. 7-9).

Step Adaptability

Optimal Client Position
Proper kinematics of the head, shoulders, and trunk; axial alignment of the shoulders, hip, knees, and ankles; pelvis rotation and kinematics; and kinematics of the hip, knee,

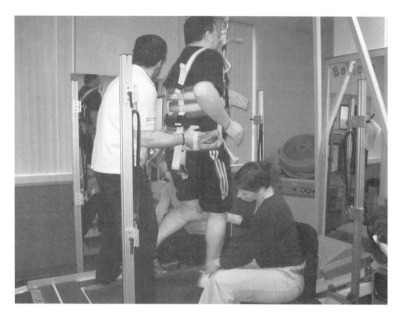

FIG 7-9 Phase 4: Step retraining. Running with <50% BWS and >3.4 mph.

and ankles during the step cycle should be maintained at pre-injury walking speeds (approximately 2.0–3.4 mph).

Trainer Instructions

The goal of step adaptability is to objectively assess independence at the trunk, pelvis, knee, and ankle during stepping. The assessment is independence at a particular BWS and speed. The recorded values are BWS and speed for independent segments. Proper kinematics of the head, shoulders, and trunk during stepping with minimal BWS and at normal walking speed is the first goal. Adding proper pelvis alignment and rotation with proper kinematics of the head, shoulders, and trunk is the second goal. Adding proper kinematics of the hip, knee, and ankle to produce flexion during swing and extension during stance and execute the stance-to-swing and swing-to-stance transitions during the step cycle form the final goal. Walking speeds and BWS are adjusted to reduce and eliminate manual facilitation during stepping at each goal. Trainers use manual facilitation as needed only at the body segments that are not the current goal for independence.

BWST Operator

Starting with the BWS and speed at the step retraining levels, treadmill speed is continuously decreased between 0.6 and 1.2 mph, and then BWS is continuously decreased to find the lowest percentage at which the client can independently maintain appropriate posture of trunk. If independence of trunk is less than 20%, BWS is increased, finding the level of independence for the pelvis. If the pelvis is independent at less than 20%, then speed is increased up to 1.9 mph. If the pelvis is still independent, then the independence of the legs is assessed and BWS is decreased with a goal of reaching below 10%, followed by increasing the speed with goal of reaching above 2.0 mph. The operator observes for appropriate posture and safety of the client while raising or lowering the support and changing the speed of the treadmill.

Hip Trainer

When specifically assessing the trunk, the trainer decreases the facilitation at the trunk while the speed is being lowered and BWS is being increased, attempting to find the highest speed and lowest BWS at which the client can maintain complete independence of the trunk with proper posture. When assessing the pelvis and legs, assistance is not provided for the trunk. When assessing the pelvis, the trainer decreases assistance at the pelvis while the speed is being lowered and BWS is being increased, attempting to find the highest speed and lowest BWS at which the client can establish complete independence of the trunk and pelvis. When assessing the legs, the trainer must not provide assistance to the trunk or pelvis.

Leg Trainers

When facilitation is needed, proper sensory cueing is used at the legs to ensure appropriate kinematics. Assistance can be provided continuously when evaluating the trunk and pelvis. When specifically assessing the legs, the trainer decreases assistance while BWS is being increased, attempting to find the highest speed and lowest BWS at which the client can establish complete independence. Both legs must be completely independent with maintained posture and position of the pelvis and extension of the hip and knee and neutral position of the ankle.

Assessment

Assessment starts with the BWS and speed at the levels at which step retraining was completed. The assessment of independence follows this order: (1) trunk, (2) hips, (3) legs. If the baseline BWS (determined during stand retraining) and speed (0.6 mph) are attained without independence for the trunk, pelvis, knee, or ankle, that particular body segment will be deemed as not attaining independence, even if independence can be attained at a higher BWS or a slower speed. First, the speed is slowed to below 1.2 mph but not lower than 0.6 mph and the BWS is increased. BWS is increased and trunk independence is evaluated. If the trunk is not independent below 20%, the actual BWS and the speed at which the trunk was independent are recorded, and then the step adaptability assessment has been completed. The pelvis is not assessed unless the trunk reaches independence below 20% with the speed between 0.6 and 1.2 mph. If the trunk and pelvis are not independent below 20%, BWS is increased continuously until the pelvis is independent. BWS is recorded and the step adaptability assessment has been completed. If the trunk and pelvis are independent below 20% BWS, treadmill speed is increased between 1.3 and 1.9 mph and then BWS is decreased to below 10%. If the trunk and pelvis are independent at below 10%, then the independence of the legs is assessed. Speed is decreased to between 0.6 and 1.2 mph; if the legs are not independent, BWS is increased. If the legs, pelvis, and trunk are independent below 10% with speeds between 1.3 and 1.9 mph, then the speed is increased toward 2.0 mph while assessing the legs. The lowest BWS and the highest speed at which the legs are independent are recorded, and the step adaptability assessment has been completed.

Scoring

- Phase 1A. Step adaptability: >60% BWS and treadmill speed 0.6–1.2 mph, unable to maintain proper kinematics of head, shoulders, and trunk. With BWS above 60% and treadmill speed between 0.6 and 1.2 mph, client still requires manual facilitation from the trainer at the head, shoulders, and/or trunk to maintain proper kinematics. Pelvis, knees, and ankles receive manual facilitation as needed.
- Phase 1B. Step adaptability: 40–59% BWS and treadmill speed 0.6–1.2 mph, maintains proper kinematics of head, shoulders, and trunk. With BWS between 40% and 59% BWS and treadmill speed between 0.6 and 1.2 mph, the client's head, shoulders, and trunk do not require manual facilitation from the trainer to maintain proper kinematics. Pelvis, knees, and ankles receive manual facilitation as needed (Fig. 7-10).
- Phase 1C. Step adaptability: 20–39% BWS and treadmill speed 0.6–1.2 mph, maintains proper kinematics of head, shoulders, and trunk. With BWS between 20% and 39% BWS and treadmill speed between 0.6 and 1.2 mph, the client's head, shoulders, and trunk do not require manual facilitation from the trainer to maintain proper kinematics. Pelvis, knees, and ankles receive manual facilitation as needed.
- Phase 2A. Step adaptability: <20% BWS and treadmill speed 0.6–1.2 mph, maintains proper kinematics of head, shoulders, and trunk. With BWS between 0% and 19% BWS and treadmill speed between 0.6 and 1.2 mph, the client's head, shoulders, and trunk do not require manual facilitation from the trainer to

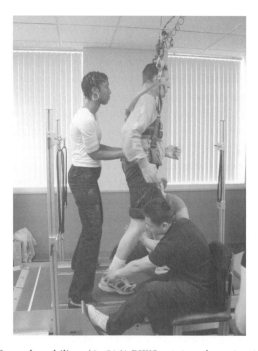

FIG 7-10 Phase 1B: Step adaptability: 40–59% BWS, <1.3 mph, maintain proper kinematics of head, shoulders, and trunk.

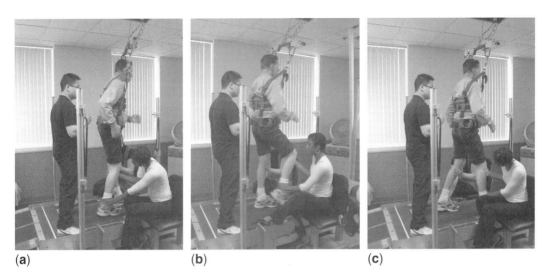

(a) **(b)** **(c)**

FIG 7-11 a, b, c. Phase 2B: Step adaptability: 40–59% BWS, <1.3 mph, maintain proper kinematics of head, shoulders, trunk, and pelvis.

maintain proper kinematics. Pelvis, knees, and ankles receive manual facilitation as needed.

- Phase 2B. Step adaptability: 40–59% BWS and treadmill speed 0.6–1.2 mph, maintains proper kinematics of head, shoulders, trunk, and pelvis. With BWS between 40% and 59% BWS and treadmill speed between 0.6 and 1.2 mph, the client's head, shoulders, and trunk do not require manual facilitation from the trainer to maintain proper kinematics. The pelvis does not need manual facilitation to maintain proper alignment, positioning, and rotation. The knees and ankles receive manual facilitation as needed (Fig. 7-11a, 7-11b, and 7-11c).

- Phase 2C. Step adaptability: 20–39% BWS and treadmill speed 0.6–1.2 mph, maintains proper kinematics of head, shoulders, trunk, and pelvis. With BWS between 20% and 39% BWS and treadmill speed between 0.6 and 1.2 mph, the client's head, shoulders, and trunk do not require manual facilitation from the trainer to maintain proper kinematics. The pelvis does not need manual facilitation to maintain proper alignment, positioning, and rotation. The knees and ankles receive manual facilitation as needed.

- Phase 3A. Step adaptability: 10–19% BWS and treadmill speed 1.3–1.9 mph, maintains proper kinematics of head, shoulders, trunk, and pelvis. With BWS between 10% and 19% BWS and treadmill speed between 1.3 and 1.9 mph, the client's head, shoulders, and trunk do not require manual facilitation from the trainer to maintain proper kinematics. The pelvis does not need manual facilitation to maintain proper alignment, positioning, and rotation. The knees and ankles receive manual facilitation as needed.

- Phase 3B. Step adaptability: <10% BWS and treadmill speed 1.3–1.9 mph, maintains proper kinematics of head, shoulders, trunk, pelvis, hips, knees, and ankles.

With BWS between 0% and 9% BWS and treadmill speed between 1.3 and 1.9 mph, the client's head, shoulders, and trunk do not require manual facilitation to maintain proper kinematics. The pelvis does not need manual facilitation to maintain proper alignment, positioning and rotation. The knees and ankles do not need manual facilitation for proper kinematics of the hips, knees, and ankles to produce the extension and flexion movements needed to complete the step cycle.

- Phase 3C. Step adaptability: <10% BWS and treadmill speed ≥2.0 mph, maintains proper kinematics of head, shoulders, trunk, pelvis, hips, knees, and ankles. With BWS between 0% and 9% BWS and treadmill speed ≥2.0 mph, the client's head, shoulders, and trunk do not require manual facilitation from the clinician to maintain proper kinematics. The pelvis does not need manual facilitation to maintain proper alignment, positioning and rotation. The knees and ankles do not need manual facilitation for proper kinematics of the hips, knees, and ankles to produce the extension and flexion movements needed to complete the step cycle.

- Phase 4. Step adaptability (running): <10% BWS and treadmill speed >3.4 mph, trunk, pelvis, and legs independent. With BWS between 0% and 9% BWS and treadmill speed >3.4 mph, the client's head, shoulders, and trunk does not require manual facilitation from the clinician to maintain proper kinematics. The pelvis does not need manual facilitation to maintain proper alignment, positioning, and rotation. The knees and ankles do not need manual facilitation for proper kinematics of the hips, knees, and ankles to produce the extension and flexion movements while being challenged with environmental adaptations and activities including running (Fig. 7-12).

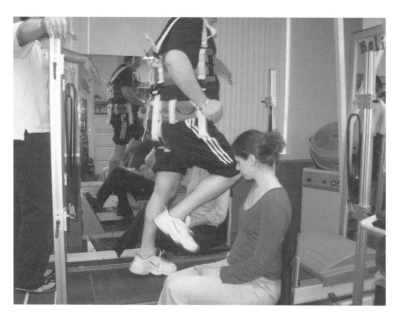

FIG 7-12 Phase 4: Step adaptability. Running with <10% BWS and >3.4 mph independent at trunk, pelvis, and legs.

Abilities During Overground Assessment

Overground assessment defines the capacity of the neuromuscular system without the benefit of the BWST or manual facilitation to execute specific motor tasks. The client is assessed beginning with Phase 1a abilities, and then assessment moves up the phase scoring. The lower phases must be achieved before higher scoring can be considered. Assistance cannot be provided to the body segment being assessed. If the client is between two phase subscores, the lower should be selected. There is no advantage to scoring higher, and all assessments should be directly compared to the pre-injury ability to complete the specific task. This is important because goal setting and progression will be based on the current phase scoring; if inappropriately scored higher, then this ability will not be sufficiently targeted for recovery during the therapeutic intervention.

Sit

Optimal Client Position
Sitting at the edge of the mat, feet flat on the floor, no upper extremity support, all with proper posture of head, shoulders, and trunk and positioning of pelvis.

Trainer Instructions
The goal is to objectively assess the level of functional recovery of sitting. With a high/low mat at a height at which the client's feet are flat on the floor, the trainer asks the client to sit up tall with his or her best attainable posture without using the hands for balance. If client cannot attain appropriate posture of the trunk, the trainer can then assist the client to the appropriate posture and then remove assistance to assess whether the client can maintain appropriate posture. If the client can maintain appropriate posture of the trunk, the trainer next assesses whether the client can attain appropriate posture of the trunk and positioning of the pelvis. If the client can indefinitely hold the position, the client is asked to sit with appropriate posture and positioning of the pelvis with arms outstretched parallel to legs. The trainer times how long the client can maintain this position. If the client maintains this position for at least 30 seconds, then he or she is asked to reach forward laterally (right and left are assessed separately) as far as possible while maintaining a steady balance. The trainer assesses the length of the forward and lateral moves. The client must be able to reach with appropriate posture and steadiness in the forward direction and on both sides. The trainer assesses whether the reaches are less than 10 or more than 10 inches. If the arms cannot reach out because of musculoskeletal dysfunction or central cord syndrome for spinal cord injury, the trainer should measure the length of movement, disregarding the inability to stretch the arm out laterally.

Scoring
- Phase 1A. Sit: Unable. Client is unable to maintain proper posture of the head, shoulders, and trunk and positioning of the pelvis during sitting. Trainers may provide manual facilitation to place the client in an appropriate sitting position. During evaluation of sitting, no manual facilitation should be provided.

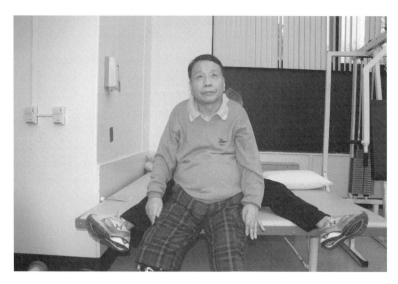

FIG 7-13 Phase 1B: Sit. Able to maintain static sitting with inappropriate posture without assist.

- Phase 1B. Sit: Unable to attain; able to sit with inappropriate posture and positioning. The client is unable to attain the position. The client is able to maintain sitting with inappropriate posture of the head, shoulders, and/or trunk and inappropriate positioning of the pelvis. Trainers may provide manual facilitation to place the client in an appropriate sitting position. During evaluation of sitting, no manual facilitation should be provided (Fig. 7-13).
- Phase 1C. Sit: unable to attain; able to sit with appropriate posture of the head, shoulders, and trunk. The client is unable to attain the position. The client is able to maintain sitting with appropriate posture of the head, shoulders, and trunk and inappropriate positioning of the pelvis. Trainers may provide manual facilitation to place the client in an appropriate sitting position. During evaluation of sitting, no manual facilitation should be provided.
- Phase 2A. Able to attain appropriate head, shoulder, and trunk posture and pelvis positioning and maintain for at least approximately 1 minute. The client is able to attain proper sitting posture and positioning from an upright position (i.e., individual is already in a sitting position and is able to attain proper head, shoulder, and trunk posture and pelvis position). The client is able to maintain sitting with appropriate posture of the head, shoulders, and trunk and proper positioning of the pelvis for approximately 1 minute. Trainers may not provide manual facilitation to place the client in an appropriate sitting position. During evaluation of sitting, no manual facilitation should be provided.
- Phase 2B. Able to attain and hold appropriate head, shoulder, and trunk posture and pelvis positioning indefinitely. The client is able to attain sitting posture and positioning from an upright position (i.e., individual is already in a sitting position

and is able to attain proper posture and pelvis position). The client is able to maintain sitting with appropriate posture of the trunk and proper positioning of the
pelvis indefinitely. Trainers may not provide manual facilitation to place the client
in an appropriate sitting posture and position. During evaluation of sitting, no
manual facilitation should be provided.

- Phase 2C. Sit with appropriate posture of the head, shoulders, and trunk and
  positioning of the pelvis with arms parallel to legs for at least 30 seconds. The client is able to attain sitting posture and positioning from an upright position (i.e.,
  individual is already in a sitting position and is able to attain proper posture and
  pelvis position). The client is able to maintain sitting with arms outstretched parallel to the legs with appropriate posture of the head, shoulders, and trunk and
  proper positioning of the pelvis for at least 30 seconds. Trainers may not provide
  manual facilitation to place the client in an appropriate sitting posture and position. During evaluation of static sitting with arms parallel, no manual facilitation
  should be provided.

- Phase 3A. Sit with proper posture of the head, shoulders, and trunk and position
  of the pelvis with forward and lateral reach <5 inches. The client is able to attain
  sitting posture and positioning from an upright position (i.e., individual is already
  in a sitting position and is able to attain proper head, shoulder, and trunk posture
  and pelvis position). The client is able to maintain sitting with appropriate posture
  of the head, shoulders, and trunk and proper positioning of the pelvis indefinitely.
  Client is able to reach forward and laterally (both right and left) less than 5 inches
  with appropriate posture of the head, shoulders, and trunk and positioning of the
  pelvis and return to the appropriate sitting posture. Trainers may not provide manual facilitation to place the client in an appropriate sitting posture and position.
  During evaluation of static sitting and reaching, no manual facilitation should be
  provided.

- Phase 3B. Sit with proper posture of the head, shoulders, and trunk and position
  of the pelvis with forward and lateral reach between approximately 5 and 10 inches.
  The client is able to attain sitting posture and positioning from an upright position (i.e., individual is already in a sitting position and is able to attain proper
  posture and pelvis position). The client is able to maintain sitting with appropriate
  posture of the head, shoulders, and trunk and proper positioning of the pelvis
  indefinitely. Client is able to maintain sitting with arms outstretched parallel to
  the legs with appropriate posture of the trunk and proper positioning of the pelvis.
  Client is able to reach forward and laterally (both right and left) between approximately 5 and 10 inches with appropriate posture of the head, shoulders, and trunk
  and positioning of the pelvis. Trainers do not provide manual facilitation for the
  head, shoulders, trunk, pelvis, hips, knees, or ankles. Trainers may not provide
  manual facilitation to place the client in an appropriate sitting posture and position. During evaluation of static sitting and reaching, no manual facilitation
  should be provided.

- Phase 3C. Sit with proper posture of the head, shoulders, and trunk and position
  of the pelvis with forward and lateral reach >10 inches. The client is able to attain
  sitting posture and positioning from an upright position (i.e., individual is already
  in a sitting position and is able to attain proper posture and pelvis position).

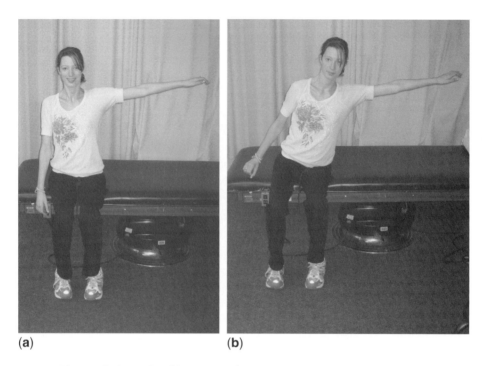

(a)   (b)

FIG 7-14 Phase 3C: Sit. **a, b.** Able to sit with appropriate posture and forward and lateral lean >10 inches and return to appropriate sitting posture.

The client is able to maintain sitting with appropriate posture of the head, shoulders, and trunk and proper positioning of the pelvis indefinitely. Client is able to maintain sitting with arms outstretched parallel to the legs with appropriate posture of the trunk and proper positioning of the pelvis. Client is able to reach forward and laterally (both right and left) greater than 10 inches with appropriate posture of the head, shoulders, and trunk and positioning of the pelvis and return to appropriate sitting posture (Fig. 7-14a and 7-14b). Trainers may not provide manual facilitation to place the client in an appropriate sitting posture and position. During evaluation of static sitting, no manual facilitation should be provided.

• Phase 4. Sit and reach: Not applicable.

Reverse Sit-Up

Optimal Client Position
Client sits on edge of mat with legs on the floor and slowly and with control lowers himself or herself onto back without use of upper extremities and maintaining knees at a 90-degree angle.

Trainer Instructions
The goal of the reverse sit-up is to objectively assess the level of functional recovery of transitioning the body from sitting to supine. With the client sitting with best attainable posture, the trainer asks the client to lower his or her trunk to the mat in a controlled manner.

The trainer should not provide assistance unless it is needed to prevent the client from striking the mat with excessive force. If the client can safely lower the trunk, the trainer first assesses the rate of movement without regard to kinematics and use of arms for counterbalance. If inappropriate kinematics are observed, the trainer verbally instructs the client to modify. If the client can control the rate of lowering the trunk, then the trainer assesses whether the client can execute the task without using the arms as a counterbalance and without extending the knees or flexing the hips. Finally, the client is asked to place his or her arms across his or her chest and perform the task again. The trainer assesses by observation and/or by asking the client how much effort was needed to execute the task.

Scoring
- Phase 1A–1C: Not applicable
- Phase 2A. Reverse sit-up: unable. Client is unable to lower his or her trunk from a sitting position to a supine position in a controlled manner with appropriate kinematics of the head, shoulders, and trunk.
- Phase 2B. Reverse sit-up: first 45 degrees. Client is able to lower his or her trunk throughout the first 45 degrees (halfway) in a controlled manner with appropriate kinematics of the head, shoulders, and trunk, but loses control during the second half (Fig. 7-15).
- Phase 2C: Not applicable
- Phase 3A. Reverse sit-up: with elevated arms and/or knee extension and/or significant hip flexion. Client is able to slowly lower his or her trunk onto the mat in a controlled manner using elevated arms to provide a counterbalance and/or knee extension and/or significant hip flexion (Fig. 7-16a, 7-16b, 7-16c).

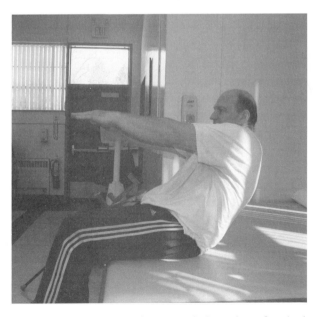

FIG 7-15 Phase 2B: Reverse sit-up. Able to lower trunk throughout first 45 degrees (halfway) in a controlled manner, but loses control during second half.

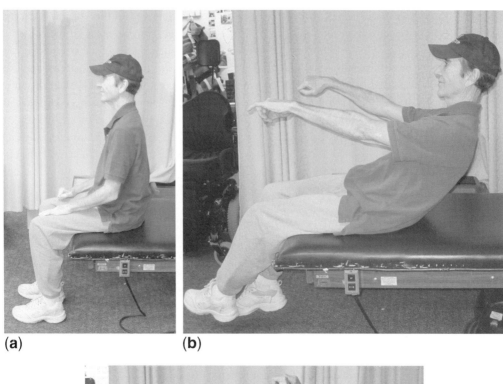

(a)   **(b)**

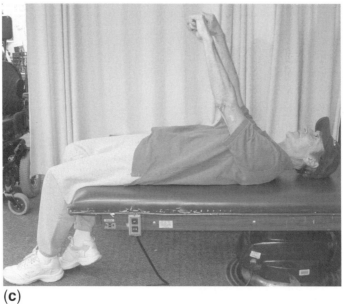

(c)

FIG 7-16 Phase 3A: Reverse sit-up. **a.** Reverse sit-up start. **b.** Midway through reverse sit-up: able to slowly lower trunk onto mat in a controlled manner using elevated arms as a counterbalance. **c.** End of reverse sit-up.

- Phase 3B: Not applicable
- Phase 3C. Reverse sit-up: with arms across chest with significant effort. With arms across chest, client is able to slowly lower his or her trunk onto the mat in a controlled manner (with appropriate kinematics of head, shoulders, trunk, and pelvis) with significant effort without knee extension or significant hip flexion.
- Phase 4. Reverse sit-up: with arms across chest without significant effort. With arms across chest, client is able to slowly lower his or her trunk onto the mat in a controlled manner with appropriate kinematics without significant effort (Fig. 7-17a, 7-17b, 7-17c).

Sit-Up

Optimal Client Position
Client lying flat on back with legs off edge of mat and comes straight up to a sitting position without use of upper extremities and maintaining knees at approximately a 90-degree angle.

Trainer Instructions
The goal of the sit-up is to objectively assess the level of functional recovery of transitioning the body from supine to sitting. With the client's feet flat on the floor and back flat against the mat, the client is asked to perform a sit-up. No manual facilitation is provided. If inappropriate kinematics are observed, the client is verbally instructed about the appropriate posture. If the client uses the momentum of arms or legs, the client is asked to repeat the sit-up and is instructed to avoid using the arms and legs. If the task is completed, the client is asked to perform the task again with arms across chest.

Scoring
- Phase 1A: Not applicable
- Phase 1B. Sit-up: unable. With shoulders in flexion, client is unable to raise his or her head off the mat.
- Phase 1C. Sit-up: raise head. With shoulders in flexion, client is able to raise his or her head off the mat (Fig. 7-18a and 7-18b).
- Phase 2A. Sit-up: raise head and initiate shoulders. With shoulders in flexion, client is able to raise his or her head and initiate raising shoulders off the mat.
- Phase 2B. Sit-up: raise head and shoulders and scapulae. With shoulders in flexion, client is able to raise his or her head and shoulders off the mat so that the inferior angles of the scapulae are off the mat (Fig. 7-19).
- Phase 2C: Not applicable
- Phase 3A. Sit-up: with elevated arms and/or knee extension and/or significant hip flexion. With shoulders in flexion, client is able to raise his or her trunk off the mat and assume a sitting position by using elevated arms to provide a counterbalance and/or knee extension and/or significant hip flexion (Fig. 7-20a and 7-20b).
- Phase 3B: Not applicable
- Phase 3C. Sit-up: with significant effort. With arms across chest, client is able to raise his or her head, shoulders, and trunk off the mat to assume sitting position with significant effort without knee extension or significant hip flexion.

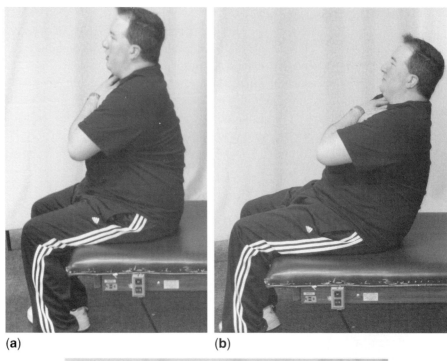

(a) (b)

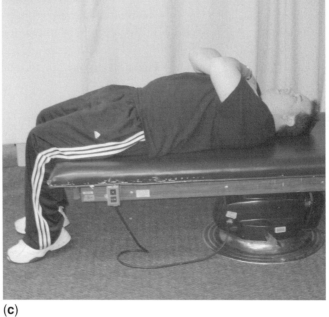

(c)

FIG 7-17 Phase 4: Reverse sit-up. With arms across chest, able to slowly lower trunk in controlled manner without significant effort. **a.** Reverse sit-up start. **b.** Midway through reverse sit-up. **c.** End of reverse sit-up.

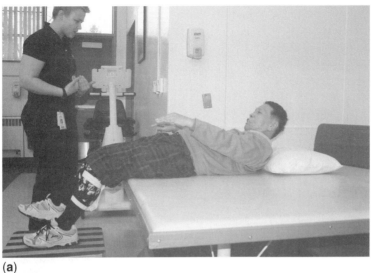

(a)

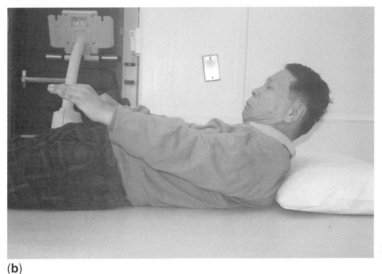

(b)

FIG 7-18 Phase 1C: Sit-up. **a, b.** With shoulders in flexion, able to raise head off mat.

- Phase 4. Sit-up: without significant effort. With arms across chest, client is able to raise head, shoulders, and trunk off the mat and assume a sitting position in a controlled manner without significant effort (Fig. 7-21a and 7-21b).

Trunk Extension in Sitting

Optimal Client Position

Client is sitting on the edge of mat with feet on the floor and chest lowered onto lap. The client slowly returns to sitting by first elevating the head and extending the neck,

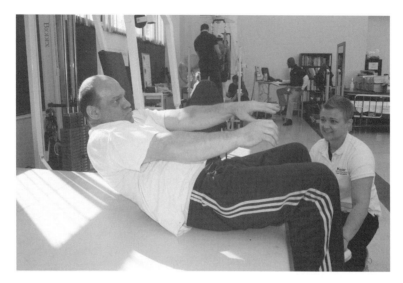

FIG 7-19 Phase 2B: Sit-up. Sit up and raise head and shoulders off mat.

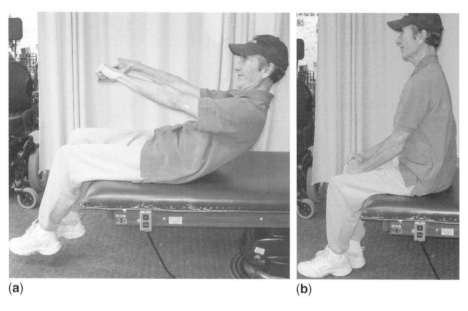

(a)   (b)

FIG 7-20 Phase 3A: Sit-up. **a.** Midway through sit-up. **b.** End of sit-up. Sit up with arms and/or knee extension and/or significant hip flexion.

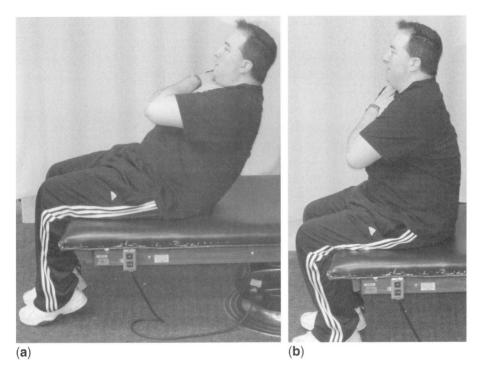

(a)   (b)

FIG 7-21 Phase 4: Sit-up. **a.** Midway through sit-up. **b.** End of sit-up. With arms across chest, the client is able to raise head, shoulders, and trunk off the mat and assume a sitting position in a controlled manner without significant effort.

then extending the shoulders and upper trunk, and finally extending the entire trunk to reach the appropriate posture and position.

Trainer Instructions

The goal of trunk extension is to objectively assess the level of functional recovery of the trunk to extend. The trainer asks the client to move into a position of sitting on the mat with chest against the quadriceps and arms hanging alongside the legs, or assists him or her into the position. No facilitation is provided during the assessment. The client is then asked to rise up to a sitting position. If the client performs this task, then the trainer asks him or her to perform it again with hands behind head. If the client performs the task with inappropriate posture and kinematics, he or she is verbally instructed to correct this and is asked to complete the task again. The trainer assesses by observation and/or by asking the client how much effort was needed to execute the task.

Scoring

- Phase 1A. Trunk extension: unable. With arms hanging down, client is unable to initiate thoracic or lumbar spine extension. Trainers may provide manual facilitation to lower the client's chest onto lap. Trainers do not provide manual facilitation for the head, shoulders, trunk, or pelvis when evaluating trunk extension.

- Phase 1B. Trunk extension: initiate thoracic spine extension. With arms hanging down, client is able to initiate thoracic spine extension. Trainers may provide manual facilitation to lower the client's chest onto lap. Trainers do not provide manual facilitation for the head, shoulders, trunk, or pelvis when evaluating trunk extension.
- Phase 1C. Trunk extension: initiate and maintain thoracic spine extension. With arms hanging down, client is able to initiate and maintain thoracic spine extension. Trainers may provide manual facilitation to lower the client's chest onto lap. Trainers do not provide manual facilitation for the head, trunk, or pelvis when evaluating trunk extension.
- Phase 2A. Trunk extension: initiate and maintain thoracic and initiate lumbar spine extension. With arms hanging down, client is able to initiate and maintain thoracic spine extension and can initiate lumbar spine extension. Trainers may provide manual facilitation to lower the client's chest onto lap. Trainers do not provide manual facilitation for the head, trunk, or pelvis when evaluating trunk extension.
- Phase 2B. Trunk extension: initiate and maintain thoracic and lumbar spine extension with significant effort. With arms hanging down, client is able to return to sitting while maintaining thoracic and lumbar spine extension with significant effort. Trainers may provide manual facilitation to lower the client's chest onto lap. Trainers do not provide manual facilitation for the head, trunk, and pelvis when evaluating trunk extension.
- Phase 2C: Not applicable
- Phase 3A. Trunk extension: initiate and maintain thoracic and lumbar spine extension without significant effort. With arms hanging down, client is able to return to sitting while maintaining lumbar and thoracic spine extension without significant effort. Trainers may provide manual facilitation to lower the client's chest onto lap. Trainers do not provide manual facilitation for the head, shoulders, trunk, and pelvis when evaluating trunk extension (Fig. 7-22a, 7-22b, 7-22c).
- Phase 3B: Not applicable
- Phase 3C. Trunk extension: hands behind head with significant effort. With hands behind his or her head, client is able to return to sitting while maintaining lumbar and thoracic spine extension with significant effort. Trainers may provide manual facilitation to lower the client's chest onto lap. Trainers do not provide manual facilitation for the head, shoulders, trunk, and pelvis when evaluating trunk extension.
- Phase 4. Trunk extension: hands behind head without significant effort. With hands behind his or her head, client is able to return to sitting while maintaining lumbar and thoracic spine extension in a controlled manner without significant effort and proper kinematics (Fig. 7-23a, 7-23b, 7-23c).

Sit to Stand

Optimal Client Position
Client sitting on edge of mat with legs on the floor steadily raises himself or herself into an upright position without use of upper extremities and with proper head, shoulder, trunk, pelvis, hip, knees, and ankle kinematics.

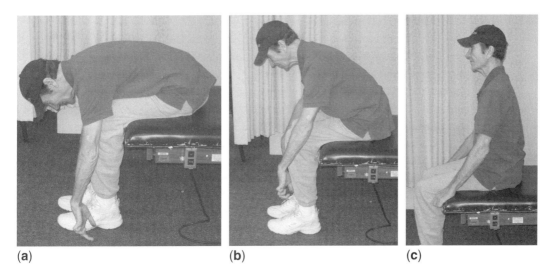

(a) (b) (c)

FIG 7-22 Phase 3A: Trunk extension in sitting. **a.** Trunk extension start. **b.** Trunk extension midway. **c.** Trunk extension end. Trunk extension: initiate and maintain thoracic and lumbar spine extension without significant effort.

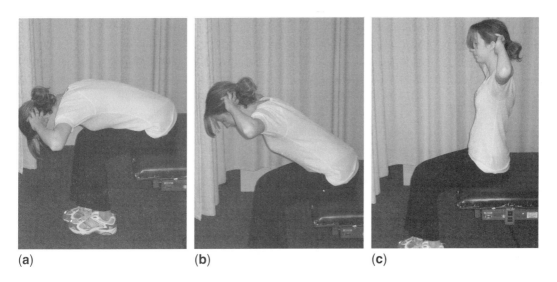

(a) (b) (c)

FIG 7-23 Phase 4: Trunk extension in sitting. **a.** Trunk extension start. **b.** Trunk extension midway. **c.** Trunk extension end. With hands behind head, able to return to sitting while maintaining lumbar and thoracic spine extension in controlled manner without significant effort.

Trainer Instructions

The goal is to objectively assess the level of functional recovery of transitioning the body from sit to stand. With the client sitting on the edge of the mat, and placing the client in the usual positioning for coming to standing, the trainer asks the client to perform a sit to stand without using hands. If the client cannot raise his or her body off the mat more than halfway, the assessment is completed. If the client can raise his or her body off the mat more than halfway but cannot completely stand up independently, the trainers may assist the pelvis and legs during the transition while first assessing the independence of the trunk. If the trunk is independent during this movement, then the transition is assessed for both trunk and pelvis and the legs can be assisted. If both the trunk and pelvis are independent during this movement, then the transition is assessed without any assistance at the trunk, pelvis, or legs. If inappropriate kinematics are observed, the trainer should verbally instruct the client. If the client is achieving sit to stand but using the arms for counterbalance, the trainer should ask him or her to attempt the movement with arms by the side.

Scoring

- Phase 1A, 1B: Not applicable
- Phase 1C. Sit to stand: unable. Client is unable to transition from sit to stand. Trainers do not provide manual facilitation for the head, shoulders, trunk, pelvis, knees, or ankles.
- Phase 2A. Sit to stand: initiate weight-bearing. Client is able to initiate weight-bearing on legs in an attempt to transition from sit to stand but unable to raise his or her body off the mat. Trainers do not provide manual facilitation for the head, shoulders, trunk, pelvis, knees, or ankles.
- Phase 2B. Sit to stand: raise body off mat <50% upright. Client is able to initiate weight-bearing on the legs and raise his or her body off the mat (less than 50% upright) during the transition from sit to stand with inappropriate kinematics of the head, shoulders, and/or trunk. Trainers do not provide manual facilitation for the head, shoulders, trunk, pelvis, knees, or ankles.
- Phase 2C. Sit to stand: maintain proper kinematics of head, shoulders, and trunk. Client is able to transition from sit to stand with appropriate kinematics of the head, shoulders, and trunk. Trainers do not provide manual facilitation for the head, shoulders, or trunk. Trainers may provide manual facilitation at the pelvis, knees, or ankles if needed.
- Phase 3A. Sit to stand: maintain proper kinematics of head, shoulders, trunk, and pelvis. Client is able to transition from sit to stand with appropriate kinematics of the head, shoulders, and trunk and positioning of the pelvis using counterbalance of arms during the transition from sit to stand. Trainers do not provide manual facilitation for the head, shoulders, trunk, or pelvis. Trainers may provide manual facilitation for knees or ankles if needed.
- Phase 3B. Sit to stand: maintain proper kinematics of head, shoulders, trunk, and pelvis with inappropriate kinematics of knees and ankles. Client is able to transition from sit to stand with appropriate kinematics of the trunk and position of the pelvis and inappropriate kinematics of the knees and ankles using counterbalance of arms during the transition from sit to stand. Trainers do not provide manual facilitation for the head, trunk, pelvis, knees, or ankles.

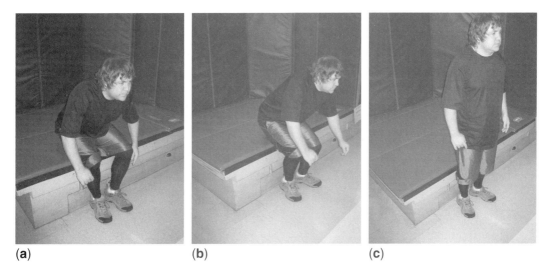

(a)   (b)   (c)

FIG 7-24 Phase 3C: Sit to stand. **a.** Sit-to-stand start. **b.** Sit-to-stand midway. **c.** Sit-to-stand end. Able to transition from sit to stand with appropriate kinematics of trunk, position of pelvis, and kinematics of legs using arms to provide counterbalance.

- Phase 3C. Sit to stand: maintain proper kinematics of head, shoulders, trunk, pelvis, knees, and ankles using arms as a counterbalance. Client is able to transition from sit to stand with appropriate kinematics of the trunk and position of the pelvis and kinematics of the knees and ankles using counter-balance of arms during the transition from sit to stand. Trainers do not provide manual facilitation for the head, trunk, pelvis, knees, or ankles (Fig. 7-24a, 7-24b, 7-24c).
- Phase 4. Sit to stand: maintain proper kinematics of head, shoulders, trunk, pelvis, knees, and ankles without using arms as a counterbalance. Client sits on edge of mat with legs on the floor and steadily raises himself or herself into an upright position with appropriate kinematics of the head, shoulders, trunk, pelvis, knees, and ankles (Fig. 7-25a, 7-25b, 7-25c). Trainers do not provide manual facilitation for the head, trunk, pelvis, knees, or ankles.

Stand

Optimal Client Position

Upright posture with the head, shoulders, and trunk extended, the pelvis properly positioned under the head and shoulders, and the knees extended to adequately maintain body weight without compensation, including hyperextension of hips and knees.

Trainer Instructions

The goal is to objectively assess the level of functional recovery of standing. With the client standing, he or she is asked to stand with his or her best attainable posture. If the

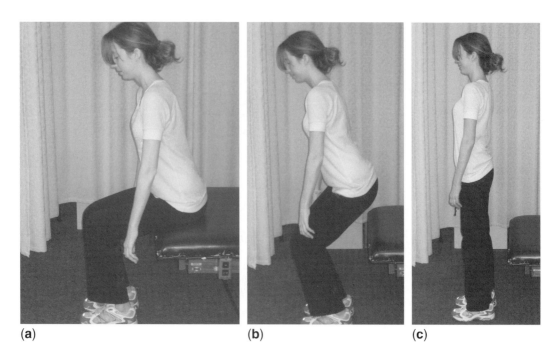

FIG 7-25 Phase 4: Sit to stand. **a.** Beginning. **b.** Midway. **c.** End position in standing. Patient sitting on mat with legs on floor steadily raises self into standing.

client cannot maintain appropriate posture, the trainers may provide assistance to the pelvis and legs If the client can maintain appropriate posture of the trunk, then the trainer assesses whether the client can attain appropriate posture of the trunk and position of the pelvis; the trainers may provide assistance to the legs. If the client can hold the position for more than a minute, then the trainer assesses whether the client can attain appropriate posture of the trunk and position of the pelvis and legs, and times how long the client can maintain this position. If the client can maintain appropriate kinematics and position indefinitely, then the trainer asks him or her to reach forward and laterally (right and left are assessed separately) as far as possible while maintaining a steady balance. The length of the lateral move is assessed. The client must be able to reach with appropriate posture and steadiness on both sides. The trainer assesses whether the reaches exceed 10 inches. If the arms cannot reach out because of musculoskeletal dysfunction or central cord syndrome for spinal cord injury, the trainer measures the length of movement disregarding the inability to stretch the arm out laterally.

Scoring

- Phase 1A, 1B: Not applicable
- Phase 1C. Stand: unable. Client is unable to maintain standing overground with proper posture of head, shoulders, and trunk and positioning of pelvis, knees, and ankles.
- Phase 2A. Stand: able to stand with inappropriate posture of the head, shoulders, and trunk. Client is able to maintain standing with inappropriate posture of

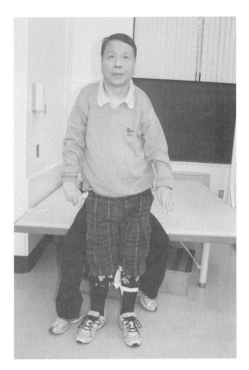

FIG 7-26 Phase 2A: Stand. Able to maintain standing with inappropriate posture of trunk.

the head, shoulders, and/or trunk. Trainers do not provide manual facilitation for the head, shoulders, or trunk. Trainers may provide manual facilitation at the pelvis, knees, or ankles as needed (Fig. 7-26).

- Phase 2B. Stand: able to stand with appropriate posture of the head, shoulders, and trunk and positioning of the pelvis for <1 minute. Client is able to maintain standing with appropriate posture of the head, shoulders, and trunk and positioning of the pelvis while using arms for a counterbalance for less than 1 minute. Trainers do not provide manual facilitation for the head, shoulders, trunk, or pelvis. Trainers may provide manual facilitation at the knees or ankles if needed.

- Phase 2C. Stand: able to stand with appropriate posture of the head, shoulders, and trunk and positioning of the pelvis for >1 minute. Client is able to maintain standing with appropriate posture of trunk and position of pelvis using the arms for a counterbalance for at least 1 minute. Trainers do not provide manual facilitation for the head, shoulders, trunk, or pelvis. Trainers may provide manual facilitation at the knees or ankles if needed.

- Phase 3A. Stand: able to stand with appropriate posture of the head, shoulders, and trunk and positioning of the pelvis, knees, and ankles for <1 minute. Client is able to maintain standing with proper posture of the trunk, position of the pelvis, and kinematics of the knees and ankles using arms for a counterbalance for less than 1 minute. Trainers do not provide manual facilitation for the head, trunk, pelvis, knees, or ankles.

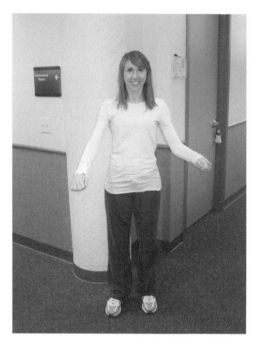

FIG 7-27 Phase 3B: Stand. Able to stand with appropriate posture of the head, shoulders, and trunk and positioning of the pelvis, knees, and ankles for >1 minute.

- Phase 3B. Stand: able to stand with appropriate posture of the head, shoulders, and trunk and positioning of the pelvis, knees, and ankles for >1 minute. Client is able to maintain standing with proper posture of the trunk, position of the pelvis, and kinematics of the knees and ankles using arms for a counterbalance for greater than 1 minute but not indefinitely. Trainers do not provide manual facilitation for the head, trunk, pelvis, knees, or ankles (Fig. 7-27).
- Phase 3C. Stand: able to stand with appropriate posture of the head, shoulders, and trunk and positioning of the pelvis, knees, and ankles indefinitely. Client is able to maintain standing with proper posture of the head, shoulders, and trunk and position of the pelvis, knees, and ankles indefinitely.

Walking

Optimal Client Position

The client is able to initiate and establish the stride position with proper kinematics and able to initiate and execute steps with head, shoulders, and trunk extended, the pelvis positioned properly under the head and shoulders, with appropriate rotation and flexion and extension of the hips, knees, and ankles at normal walking speed.

Trainer Instructions

The goal is to objectively assess the level of functional recovery of walking. With client in standing position, the trainer asks the client to weight shift side to side. If the client cannot shift the weight laterally, the trainers may provide manual facilitation at the hips and legs for balance but should not assist in shifting of the weight. If the client can shift the weight laterally with appropriate kinematics of the trunk, then the client is asked to get into a stride position and shift weight back and forth. The trainer may assist the client into the stride position since the assessment is now only on ability to shift weight back and forth in the stride position. This should be tested both with the right and left legs forward. If the client can maintain appropriate kinematics of the trunk, the client is asked to move to a stand position and shift weight laterally and then move into a stride position and shift weight back and forth in the stride position with appropriate kinematics of the trunk and legs. The trainer can manually facilitate at the hips but should not assist the trunk or legs. If the client can shift weight in all directions with appropriate kinematics at the trunk and legs, the client is asked to take several consecutive steps. Manual facilitation should not be provided for the trunk, pelvis, or legs. If inappropriate kinematics are observed, the trainer should verbally instruct the client to modify.

Scoring

- Phase 1A–2C: Not applicable
- Phase 2A. Lateral (side to side): unable. Client is unable to shift body weight laterally (side to side).
- Phase 2B. Lateral (side to side): weight shift with inappropriate head, shoulder, and trunk kinematics. The client is able to shift body weight laterally (side to side) with inappropriate kinematics of head, shoulders, and/or trunk. Trainers do not provide manual facilitation for the head, shoulders, or trunk. Trainers may provide manual facilitation at the pelvis, knees, and/or ankles if needed.
- Phase 2C. Lateral (side-to-side) and in-stride (back-and-forth) weight shift with appropriate kinematics of head, shoulders, and trunk. The client is able to shift body weight laterally (side to side) with appropriate kinematics of head, shoulders, and trunk. Client is unable to initiate the stride position with the right and/or left leg forward. Trainers may provide manual facilitation to achieve the proper stride position. The client is able to shift weight in the stride position (back and forth) with appropriate kinematics of head, shoulders, and trunk. Trainers do not provide manual facilitation for the head, shoulders, or trunk during weight shifts in the lateral and stride positions.
- Phase 3A. Lateral (side-to-side) and in-stride (back-and-forth) weight shift with appropriate kinematics of head, shoulders, and trunk and inappropriate kinematics of the legs. The client is able to shift body weight laterally (side to side) at the trunk with appropriate kinematics of the head, trunk, and shoulders and with inappropriate kinematics of the knees and ankles. Client is able to initiate and complete the stride position with both the right and left leg forward and is able to shift weight in the stride position (back and forth) with appropriate kinematics of the head, shoulders, and trunk. Trainers do not provide manual facilitation for the head, trunk, knees, or ankles to achieve the proper stride position or during weight shifts. Trainers may provide manual facilitation at the pelvis to achieve the proper stride position and during weight shifts in the lateral and stride positions. The client may make several attempts at achieving the stride position, including several small steps and repositioning of the ankle and foot to achieve the proper stride position.

- Phase 3B. Lateral (side-to-side) and in-stride (back and forth) weight shift with appropriate kinematics of head, shoulders, trunk, knee, and ankle. Client is able to shift body weight laterally (side to side) at the trunk with appropriate kinematics of the head, shoulders, knees, and ankles. Client is able to initiate and complete the stride position both with the right and left leg forward with appropriate kinematics at the head, shoulders, trunk, knees, and ankles and is able to shift weight in the stride position (back and forth) with appropriate kinematics of the head, shoulders, and trunk. Trainers do not provide manual facilitation for the head, shoulders, trunk, knees, or ankles to achieve the proper stride position or during weight shifts in the lateral and stride positions. Trainers may provide manual facilitation at the pelvis to achieve the proper stride position and during weight shifts in the lateral and stride positions (Fig. 7-28a and 7-28b).
- Phase 3C. Repetitive steps with appropriate kinematics of head, shoulders, and trunk. Client is able to shift body weight laterally (side to side) AND able to shift weight in stride position (back and forth) with appropriate kinematics of the head, shoulders, trunk, and legs. Client is able to initiate a step with both the left and right leg and continue with repetitive steps with appropriate kinematics of the head, shoulders, and trunk and with inappropriate kinematics of the pelvis, knees, and/or ankles (Fig. 7-29a, 7-29b, 7-29c). Trainers should not provide manual facilitation to the trunk, pelvis, or legs.

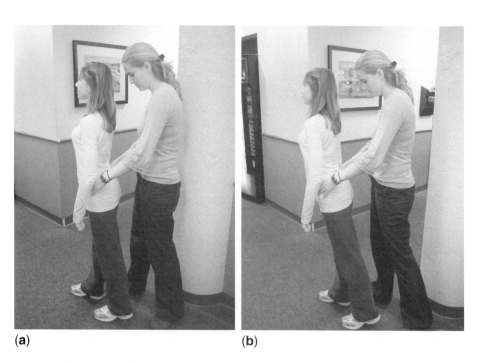

(a)　　　　　　　　　　　　　**(b)**

FIG 7-28 Phase 3B: Walking: Weight shift. **a.** Beginning of stride weight shift. **b.** End of stride weight shift. Able to shift body weight laterally and back and forth with appropriate posture and kinematics at the legs. Able to initiate and complete stride position with appropriate posture at trunk and kinematics at the legs.

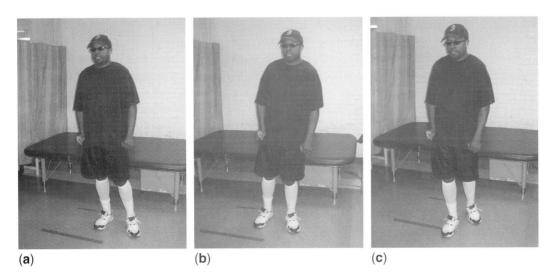

(a)   (b)   (c)

FIG 7-29 Phase 3C: Walking. Weight shift. Able to continue with repetitive steps **a.** Able to shift body weight laterally. **b.** Able to shift body weight laterally. **c.** Stride weight shift with repetitive steps.

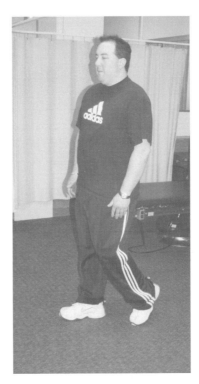

FIG 7-30 Phase 4: Walking. Same as 3C and able to continue with repetitive steps with appropriate kinematics at trunk, pelvis, and legs.

- Phase 4. Walking with appropriate kinematics of head, shoulders, trunk, pelvis, and legs. Client is able to shift body weight laterally (side to side) AND able to shift weight back and forth in the stride position independently at the trunk with appropriate posture and independently at the pelvis and legs with appropriate kinematics. Client is able to initiate and complete the stride position independently with appropriate kinematics at the trunk, pelvis, and legs. Client is able to continue with repetitive steps with appropriate kinematics at the trunk, pelvis, and legs (Fig. 7-30). Trainers should not provide manual facilitation to the trunk, pelvis, or legs.

Overview of Utilization of Phases of Recovery for Progression

The trainer should calculate the overall phase number (see phase sheets, Appendix A) after completing the assessments. The complete phase assessment should be conducted approximately every 20 sessions to monitor the recovery progress of the client and set overall intervention goals. We recommend continuing the intervention as long as the individual has improved in at least one task by one subphase (e.g., moving from Phase 1A to Phase 1B). This includes abilities during step training or any task during the over-ground assessment. The three tasks that score the lowest should be assessed daily during the overground assessment component of the therapy to monitor short-term progress and prioritize goals. The next chapter discusses specific recommendations for the progression of the client toward full recovery.

Appendix A

Phase Scoring Sheet

Stand Retraining	Stand Adaptability	Step Retraining	Step Adaptability	Sit	Reverse Sit Up	Sit Up	Trunk Extension	Sit to Stand	Stand	Walking
1A	1A	1A	1A	1A	1A	1A	1A	1A	1A	1A
1B	1B	1B	1B	1B	1B	1B	1B	1B	1B	1B
1C	1C	1C	1C	1C	1C	1C	1C	1C	1C	1C
2A	2A	2A	2A	2A	2A	2A	2A	2A	2A	2A
2B	2B	2B	2B	2B	2B	2B	2B	2B	2B	2B
2C	2C	2C	2C	2C	2C	2C	2C	2C	2C	2C
3A	3A	3A	3A	3A	3A	3A	3A	3A	3A	3A
3B	3B	3B	3B	3B	3B	3B	3B	3B	3B	3B
3C	3C	3C	3C	3C	3C	3C	3C	3C	3C	3C
4	4	4	4	4	4	4	4	4	4	4

Patient ID:	Left Leg				Right Leg			
Date:	Flexor	High	Mod	Low	Flexor	High	Mod	Low
Center:	Extensor	High	Mod	Low	Extensor	High	Mod	Low
Overall Phase:	Predominant overall pattern	Flex > Ext	Balanced	Ext > Flex	Predominant overall pattern	Flex > Ext	Balanced	Ext > Flex

Appendix B

Phase Sheet Cards

Stand Adaptability

1A With >60% BWS, unable to maintain proper posture at trunk.

2A With 0-19% BWS, able to maintain proper posture at trunk.

3A NOT APPLICABLE

1B With 40-59% BWS, able to maintain proper posture at trunk.

2B With 40-59% BWS, able to maintain proper posture at trunk & position of pelvis.

3B With <10% BWS, able to maintain proper posture at trunk & position of pelvis.

1C With 20-39% BWS, able to maintain proper posture at trunk.

2C With 10-39% BWS, able to maintain proper posture at trunk & position of pelvis.

3C With <10% BWS, able to maintain proper posture at trunk & position of pelvis & legs. BWS may be used as safety for balance deficiencies.

4 With 0% BWS, able to maintain proper posture at trunk & position of pelvis & legs & balance.

Step Retraining

1A BWS must be >60% to generate best stepping pattern. At BWS 60% or below, trainers are unable to maintain proper kinematics.

2A Able to generate best stepping pattern at 45-49% BWS. At BWS 44% or below, trainers are unable to maintain proper kinematics.

3A Able to generate best stepping pattern at 30-34% BWS. At BWS 29% or below, trainers are unable to maintain proper kinematics.

1B Able to generate best stepping pattern at 55-59% BWS. At BWS 54% or below, trainers are unable to maintain proper kinematics.

2B Able to generate best stepping pattern at 40-44% BWS. At BWS 39% or below, trainers are unable to maintain proper kinematics.

3B Able to generate best stepping pattern at 20-29% BWS. At BWS 19% or below, trainers are unable to maintain proper kinematics.

1C Able to generate best stepping pattern at 50-54% BWS. At BWS 49% or below, trainers are unable to maintain proper kinematics.

2C Able to generate best stepping pattern at 35-39% BWS. At BWS 34% or below, trainers are unable to maintain proper kinematics.

3C Able to generate best stepping pattern at 0-19% BWS and maintain proper kinematics.

4 Able to generate a stepping/running pattern between 0-49% BWS & over 3.4 mph (as in running) with proper kinematics.

Stand Retraining

1A Able to maintain proper posture of trunk, position of pelvis and legs at ? 40% BWS with trainer assist for at least 5 min.

2A NOT APPLICABLE

3A NOT APPLICABLE

1B Able to maintain proper posture of trunk & position of pelvis and legs at 20-39% BWS with trainer assist for at least 5 min.

2B Able to maintain proper posture of trunk & position of pelvis and legs at 10-19% BWS with trainer assist for at least 5 min.

3B NOT APPLICABLE

1C NOT APPLICABLE

2C NOT APPLICABLE

3C Able to maintain proper posture of trunk and position of pelvis and legs at 0-9% BWS with trainer assist for at least 5 min.

4 NOT APPLICABLE

Step Adaptability

1A With BWS >60% & treadmill speed 0.6-1.2 mph, unable to maintain proper kinematics.

IB With BWS 40-59% & treadmill speed 0.6-1.2 mph, able to maintain proper trunk kinematics.

1C With BWS 20-39% & treadmill speed 0.6-1.2 mph, able to maintain proper trunk kinematics.

2A With BWS <20% & treadmill speed 0.6-1.2 mph, able to maintain proper trunk kinematics.

2B With BWS 40-59% & treadmill speed 0.6-1.2 mph, able to maintain proper trunk and pelvis kinematics.

2C With BWS 20-39% & treadmill speed 0.6-1.2 mph, able to maintain proper trunk and pelvis kinematics.

3A With BWS <20% & treadmill speed 1.3-1.9 mph, able to maintain proper trunk and pelvis kinematics.

3B With BWS <10% & treadmill speed 1.3-1.9 mph, able to maintain proper trunk, pelvis and leg kinematics.

3C With BWS <10% & treadmill speed >2.0 mph, able to maintain proper trunk, pelvis and leg kinematics.

4 With BWS <10% & treadmill speed >3.4 mph, able to maintain proper trunk, pelvis and leg kinematics.

Reverse Sit Up

1A NOT APPLICABLE

IB NOT APPLICABLE

1C NOT APPLICABLE

2A Unable to lower trunk in a controlled manner.

2B Able to lower trunk throughout first 45 degrees (1/2 way) in a controlled manner, but loses control during 2nd half.

2C NOT APPLICABLE

3A Able to slowly lower trunk onto mat in a controlled manner using elevated arms to provide a counter-balance &/or knee extension &/or significant hip flexion.

3B NOT APPLICABLE

3C With arms across chest, able to slowly lower trunk onto mat in a controlled manner with significant effort without knee extension or significant hip flexion.

4 With arms across chest, able to slowly lower trunk onto mat in a controlled manner without significant effort.

Sit Up

1A NOT APPLICABLE

1B With shoulders in flexion, unable to raise head off of mat.

1C With shoulders in flexion, able to raise head off of mat.

2A With shoulders in flexion, able to raise head & initiate raising shoulders off of mat.

2B With shoulders in flexion, able to raise head & shoulders off of mat so that inferior angles of scapulae are off of mat.

2C NOT APPLICABLE

3A With shoulders in flexion, able to raise trunk off of mat & assume a sitting position by using elevated arms to provide a counter-balance &/or knee extension &/or significant hip flexion.

3B NOT APPLICABLE

3C With arms across chest, able to raise head, shoulders & trunk off of mat to assume sitting position with significant effort without knee extension or significant hip flexion.

4 With arms across chest, able to raise head, shoulders & trunk off of mat & assume sitting position in a controlled manner without significant effort.

Sit

1A Unable to maintain proper posture of trunk and position of pelvis.

1B Unable to attain. Able to maintain sitting with inappropriate posture of trunk and inappropriate position of pelvis.

1C Unable to attain. Able to maintain sitting with appropriate posture of trunk and inappropriate position of pelvis.

2A Able to both attain sitting with appropriate posture of trunk and position of pelvis & maintain this for approx. one min.

2B Able to both attain sitting with appropriate posture of trunk and position of pelvis & maintain this indefinitely.

2C Able to both attain sitting with appropriate posture of trunk and position of pelvis with arms outstretched parallel to the legs for at least 30 sec.

3A Able to attain & maintain appropriate sitting posture indefinitely, to elevate arms outstretched parallel to legs & forward & lateral reach/lean <5 inches & return to appropriate sitting posture.

3B Able to attain & maintain appropriate sitting posture indefinitely. Able to elevate arms out-stretched parallel to legs & forward and lateral reach/lean 5-10 inches & return to appropriate sitting posture.

3C Able to attain & maintain appropriate sitting posture indefinitely. Able to forward & lateral reach/lean >10 inches & return to appropriate sitting posture.

4 NOT APPLICABLE

Trunk Extension in Sitting

1A With arms hanging down, unable to initiate thoracic spine extension.

1B With arms hanging down, able to initiate thoracic spine extension.

1C With arms hanging down, able to initiate & maintain thoracic spine extension.

2A With arms hanging down, able to initiate & maintain thoracic spine extension & can initiate lumbar spine extension.

2B With arms hanging down, able to return to sitting while maintaining thoracic & lumbar spine extension with significant effort.

2C NOT APPLICABLE

3A With arms hanging down, able to return to sitting while maintaining lumbar & thoracic spine extension without significant effort.

3B NOT APPLICABLE

3C With hands behind head, able to return to sitting while maintaining lumbar & thoracic spine extension with significant effort.

4 With hands behind head, able to return to sitting while maintaining lumbar & thoracic spine extension in controlled manner without significant effort.

Stand

1A NOT APPLICABLE

IB NOT APPLICABLE

1C Unable to maintain standing overground with proper posture of trunk and position of pelvis and legs.

2A Able to maintain standing with inappropriate posture of trunk.

2B Able to maintain standing with appropriate posture of trunk & position of pelvis using arms for counter balance for <1 min.

2C Able to maintain standing with appropriate posture of trunk & position of pelvis using arms for a counter balance for at least one min.

3A Able to maintain standing with proper trunk posture & position of pelvis and legs using arms for a counter balance for <1 min.

3B Able to maintain standing with proper trunk posture & position of pelvis and legs using arms for a counter balance for >1 min, but not indefinitely.

3C Able to maintain standing with proper trunk posture & position of pelvis and legs indefinitely.

4 Able to maintain standing with proper trunk posture & position of pelvis & legs & reach/lean with arms in all directions >10 in.

Walking

1A NOT APPLICABLE

2A Unable to shift body weight laterally (side to side).

3A Able to shift body wt laterally & able to shift wt back & forth in stride position with appropriate posture at trunk & inappropriate kinematics at legs. Able to initiate & complete stride position with appropriate posture at trunk & inappropriate kinematics at legs.

IB NOT APPLICABLE

2B Able to shift body wt laterally (side to side) with inappropriate kinematics at trunk.

3B Able to shift body wt laterally & able to shift wt back & forth in stride position with appropriate posture at trunk and appropriate kinematics at legs. Able to initiate and complete stride position with appropriate posture at trunk and with appropriate kinematics at legs.

1C NOT APPLICABLE

2C Able to shift body wt laterally with appropriate kinematics at trunk. Able to weight shift back and forth with appropriate kinematics at the trunk.

3C SAME AS 3B plus able to continue with repetitive steps with appropriate kinematics at trunk, and inappropriate kinematics at pelvis and legs.

4 SAME AS 3B plus able to continue with repetitive steps with appropriate kinematics at trunk, pelvis and legs.

Sit to Stand

1A NOT APPLICABLE

2A Able to initiate weight bearing in an attempt to transition from sit to stand but unable to raise body off of mat.

3A Able to transition from sit to stand with appropriate kinematics at trunk & position of pelvis using counter balance of arms.

IB NOT APPLICABLE

2B Able to initiate weight bearing on legs & raise body off of mat (less than 50% upright) during transition from sit to stand.

3B Able to transition from sit to stand with appropriate kinematics at trunk and position of pelvis and inappropriate kinematics at legs using counter balance of arms.

1C Unable to transition from sit to stand.

2C Able to transition from sit to stand with appropriate kinematics of trunk.

3C Able to transition from sit to stand with appropriate kinematics of trunk, position of pelvis, and kinematics of legs using arms to provide counter balance.

4 Patient sitting on edge of mat with legs on floor steadily raises self into an upright position.

Calculate Overall Phase

1. Rate each item (Stand Retraining, Sit Up, Stand, etc.) using the definitions on the other cards.

2. To calculate the overall score, you'll need to find the item with the lowest phase rating and one or two phases higher than the lowest phase rating. Example: if the lowest phase = 1C, one phase higher than the lowest phase = 2A, two phases higher than the lowest phase = 2B.

3. Calculate the overall score:

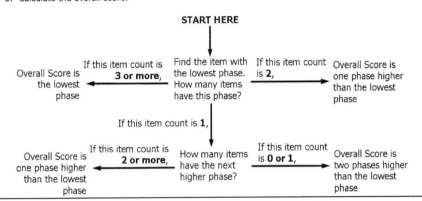

8

Progression to Recovery

Chapter Outline

D. Phase 4 Progression
      i. Step Training
      ii. Overground Assessment
      iii. Community Integration
III. Overall Summary

Chapter Objectives

The objectives of Chapter 8 are to:

1. Define the four areas of progression.
2. Describe key means of progression by phase of neuromuscular recovery (Phases 1, 2, 3, and 4) and by the three components of Locomotor Training (step retraining, overground assessment, and community integration).
3. Describe the change in emphasis for progression within step training for stand and step retraining and for stand and step adaptability as the client recovers.

Summary

Properly and continuously challenging clients to achieve higher levels of performance is critical to recovery. Therapists and technicians must know how to use progression strategies for each phase if they are to optimize recovery and assist the client on the road to recovery. Four areas of progression (endurance, speed, load, and independence) are emphasized based on the phase of recovery the client is experiencing. The physical therapist should closely monitor those tasks that are scored the lowest during phasing and target their specific goals and clinical decision making to help the client move to the next level.

Four Areas of Progress

The rate and extent of recovery will be related to the level at which the therapeutic intervention challenges the neuromuscular system. The four critical areas of progression are (1) endurance, (2) speed, (3) loading, and (4) independence. Areas of progression can be challenged simultaneously. Trainers may have to compromise one area of progression to address another and then return to the initial area to regain that level of ability. For example, weight-bearing on the legs may need to be decreased (by increasing body weight support) to increase speed or gain independence. The order of progression is prioritized and for retraining is (1) speed, (2) endurance, (3) loading, and (4) independence. In comparison, the order of progression is prioritized for adaptability and is (1) independence, (2) loading, (3) speed, and (4) endurance. These progression goals are also implemented in parallel in the community integration component. The clinician is constantly making decisions regarding progression throughout the activity-based rehabilitation program.

Endurance

Endurance is generally defined as the amount of time an individual can continuously execute a task. This can be applied to all of the components of Locomotor Training. During step training endurance includes the total length of time an individual is able to bear weight using body weight support on the treadmill (BWST), the length of time he or she can continuously stand or step retrain, as well as the length of time he or she can step or stand independently on the treadmill.

When initiating the Locomotor Training intervention the BWS and speed should be adjusted to reach 60 minutes of total weight-bearing, including step retraining, stand retraining, step adaptability, and stand adaptability. For step retraining the first goal is to achieve a minimum of 20 minutes of step retraining time at normal walking speeds, and the BWS is adjusted accordingly. Repetition and practice intensity is necessary to achieve a therapeutic effect. After this is achieved, then BWS can be lowered. If the client requires stand training, then BWS should be adjusted to maintain a 5-minute bout. After this is achieved, then BWS can be lowered. When defining the step training session, stepping should occur longer than standing, and retraining should occur longer than adaptability for both stepping and standing.

For stand and step adaptability, endurance is a focus in the later stages of recovery. Endurance can also be challenged in the overground environment with community integration during mobility, transitions, sitting, standing, and walking. Endurance can be increased by advising the client to practice specific tasks at home and gradually increasing the number of repetitions and/or continuous time executing the task.

Speed

Challenging speed occurs during step training, step adaptability, and walking overground. During step training, the evidence suggests that optimal retraining occurs during normal walking speeds (see Chapter 2). Thus, during step training bouts, the treadmill speed should be the first parameter optimized. Achieving normal walking speed will be prioritized over increasing load; thus, BWS should be adjusted to maintain normative walking speeds while trainers provide manual facilitation as needed.

During step adaptability the focus is independence, and the clinician should continuously challenge the independence of the neuromuscular system to stand and step without manual facilitation. Increasing the stepping speed can promote appropriate intralimb and interlimb coordination and appropriate kinematics at the trunk, pelvis, and lower limbs but is progressed only after full weight-bearing has been achieved. During community integration, the clinician should select assistive devices that can be used to promote the overground practice of speed.

Load

Increasing the ability to load (bear weight) is important both for retraining the nervous system and for achieving independence of standing and walking overground. During stand training, decreasing the level of BWS to maximize the loading on the legs should be the first parameter implemented, with manual facilitation provided to maintain the proper posture and positioning. During step training, increasing the load will provide higher levels of activation (but should be challenged without reducing the speed of stepping). During step and stand adaptability the load should be challenged first (prior to increasing the speed) by decreasing the BWS, but not at the expense of allowing the independence for the targeted body segment from manual facilitation. Whenever weight-bearing is possible it should be elicited during community integration. The client should be encouraged to bear weight on the legs and stand whenever possible in the home and community.

Independence

Independence is the ultimate goal desired by the client. It can be defined in many ways within Locomotor Training, including independence from (1) manual facilitation at the trunk, hip, and legs, (2) BWS during step training, (3) bungees during stepping, (4) braces, and (5) assistive devices. Independence is first progressed during stand and step adaptability and then correspondingly during community integration. Independence is the first goal while BWS and speed are adjusted to allow independent trunk, pelvis, and leg control by the individual. The progression of independence is sequenced by first progressing the trunk, then the pelvis, and finally the legs. This approach is additive in that once the trunk is independent and the focus is on the independence of the pelvis, the trunk must also be independent as well. Correspondingly, when the legs are progressed, this would be with both the trunk and pelvis independent. The trainers must not provide assistance for the trunk and pelvis or the legs at all when this is the focus of the adaptability session and normal kinematics is not necessarily expected. When challenging the neuromuscular system, BWS should be lowered prior to increasing speed so that overground walking can be initiated at the earliest time.

Community integration transfers the capacity that is developed by retraining and challenged during adaptability into functional goals in the home and community. Trainers should identify the areas where independence can be introduced into functional goals and daily activities. Trainers should select the least restrictive assistive device and avoid or eliminate bracing as soon as possible to promote independence and always have times when the current goal is practiced without any compensation. The client is encouraged to execute movements with the kinematics used pre-injury whenever possible.

Progression by Phase of Recovery and Locomotor Training Component

Phase 1 Progression

Clients in Phase 1 of recovery most benefit by receiving the Locomotor Training intervention five times per week to provide intense retraining of the nervous system. Clients in the earliest phase of recovery may have impairments in cardiovascular and pulmonary function, poor circulation and temperature control, spasticity that interferes with sleep and/or daily function, atrophied muscles, decreased bone density, and pressure sores. These conditions may be in part attributable to their need for maximal assistance for mobility and their inability to bear weight, stand, and walk. The focus of Locomotor

Training for these individuals is to increase weight-bearing (standing and stepping), improve endurance, and improve posture and strength of the neck, shoulders, and trunk. These primary goals are implemented in each component of Locomotor Training, including step training (retraining and adaptability), overground assessment (adaptability), and community integration (adaptability).

Step Training

Phase 1 step training emphasizes step and stand retraining while increasing endurance. The total time stepping and standing should reach 1 continuous hour per session as soon as possible. Four skilled trainers are usually needed to implement the treatment intervention properly, as clients generally need assistance at all three body segments (both legs and trunk/pelvis), and clients and trainers need feedback from an involved BWST operator to maintain an optimal standing posture and stepping pattern. The Locomotor Training sessions should include clear and concise instructions to the client. By providing explicit directions and basic education in the Locomotor Training principles and proper techniques, the client is encouraged to become an active participant in recovery.

As the primary emphasis in Phase 1 is on retraining the neuromuscular system, about 75% of the total training time focuses on retraining and about 25% emphasizes adaptability (Fig. 8-1, top). The 75% retraining time should be divided between step retraining and stand retraining, with step training occurring for 20 to 30 minutes (Fig. 8-1, middle). The 25% adaptability should be divided with a greater proportion of time targeting stand adaptability (about 20%) compared to about 5% with step adaptability (Fig. 8-1, bottom). In all sessions, the time spent stepping should always be greater than standing; and the time spent step retraining should always be greater than step adaptability.

Step retraining emphasizes increasing endurance during stepping at normal walking speeds while achieving proper kinematics with manual facilitation at the trunk, pelvis, knees, and ankles as needed. BWS is lowered as tolerated by the client and trainers. Therefore, retraining will focus on establishing good stepping at a normal walking speed and decreasing the BWS as tolerated by the client and trainers. Stand retraining goals focus on endurance (total time standing) and maximally loading during upright standing, with trainers providing manual facilitation to maintain proper posture, alignment, and joint positions as needed. Step adaptability focuses on trunk independence. Stepping speed is adjusted to lower speeds and BWS is increased to allow optimization of independence of the trunk while increasing endurance, and then progressed over time by lowering the BWS. Stand adaptability focuses on independence from manual facilitation at the head, shoulders, and trunk while increasing weight-bearing. The trainer can ask the client to lean forward and initiate trunk extension back to an upright position (Fig. 8-2a and 8-2b). Arm strengthening during standing may also be incorporated during the stand adaptability bout, but manual facilitation to the trunk should not be provided.

Overground Assessment

Daily overground assessment in Phase 1 focuses primarily on head, shoulder, and trunk independence during sitting, position changes from supine to sitting, and trunk extension. Each session, the physical therapist should assess the three lagging items, which most often involve the ability to sit, maintain trunk stability, and flex and extend the trunk, and then focus community integration activities on achieving the next level

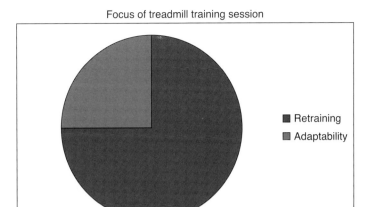

Focus of treadmill training session

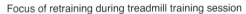

Focus of retraining during treadmill training session

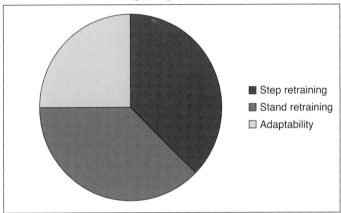

Focus of adaptability during treadmill training session

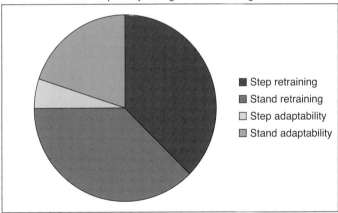

FIG 8-1 Phase 1: Approximate proportions of time spent in a training session on retraining (step and stand) and adaptability (step and stand).

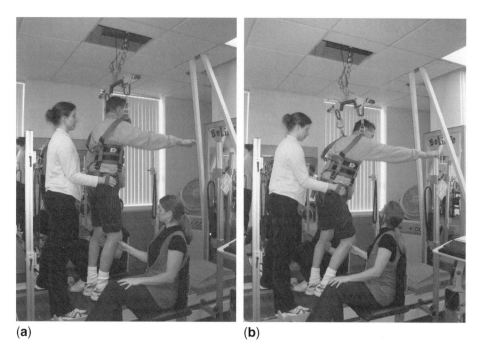

(a)   **(b)**

FIG 8-2 a, b. Phase 1: Stand adaptability progression. Forward reaching.

of ability. The therapist assesses the client's ability, identifies the limiting factor to move forward to the next level of recovery (subphase), and makes decisions about goals for the next step training session as well as recommendations for community integration.

Community Integration

Community integration goals in Phase 1 focus on trunk activation and appropriate posture during sitting, position changes from supine to sitting, wheelchair propulsion, transfers, and other activities. Home exercises in community integration should focus on strengthening of core trunk muscles that target promoting independent bed mobility, trunk stability during position changes and sitting, independent transfers, and the use of a manual wheelchair, if not already used. Any activities that can load the legs, such as practicing shifting weight onto the legs during sitting or during transfers, should be encouraged. Strengthening exercises such as trunk extensions and partial sit-ups should be done at home. Family support during this phase is critical, as assistance may be required to promote such experiences.

Phase 2 Progression

Clients in Phase 2 of recovery benefit by receiving Locomotor Training a minimum of four times per week (clients should be encouraged to maintain 5 days per week until reaching a Phase 2b classification because regression or plateaus may occur) to repetitively reinforce the presentation of sensory cues during walking, with emphasis on challenging both the trunk and pelvis to be independent during position changes, sitting, standing, and walking. Clients in the mid-stage of recovery may have achieved independence in supine and sitting mobility and transfers but are not able to transition from sit to stand, stand, or walk independently. The focus of Locomotor Training for these individuals is to increase independent weight-bearing and improve proper positioning of the pelvis during sitting and standing and appropriate trunk kinematics during the transition from sit to stand and during weight shifting. These primary goals are implemented in each component of Locomotor Training, including step training (retraining and adaptability), overground assessment (adaptability), and community integration (adaptability).

Step Training

Clients progressing to Phase 2 usually have the endurance to maintain 1 hour of step training, and the emphasis is on retraining while decreasing BWS to maximize loading on the legs. Four skilled trainers (including the BWST operator) are generally required to implement the treatment intervention properly, since clients should be independent at the trunk but may need assistance at the pelvis and legs for a majority of the step training session (Fig. 8-3a–d). Step training emphasizes maintaining endurance at normal walking speeds while increasing the load on the legs (decreasing BWS) and achieving trunk/pelvis independence.

As the goals shift from Phase 1 to Phase 2, the proportion of time in stand retraining is reduced while the proportion of adaptability is increased during a step training session. In Phase 2, about 60% of the total training time is retraining, while about 40% targets adaptability (Fig. 8-4, top). The 60% retraining time is divided with about 55% for step retraining and about 5% in stand retraining (Fig. 8-4, middle). The client is now spending more time in standing at home, so the efforts in retraining concentrate on step retraining. The 40% adaptability is with a greater proportion of time targeting stand adaptability (about 20%) compared to about 5% with step adaptability (Fig. 8-4, bottom).

Step retraining emphasizes decreasing BWS at normal walking speeds and achieving proper kinematics with manual facilitation at the trunk, pelvis, knees, and ankles as needed. BWS is lowered whenever possible while still maintaining a good stepping pattern until the client is bearing a majority of his or her weight (≤40% BWS). Stand retraining goals focus on reducing the BWS to reach full weight-bearing during upright standing, with trainers providing manual facilitation to maintain proper posture, alignment, and kinematics. Stand retraining is no longer needed when the trunk has achieved independence with BWS below 10%. Step adaptability focuses on trunk independence at less than 25% BWS and proper pelvis positioning during stepping with BWS from 25% to 49%. Speeds remain lower to allow independence at the trunk and pelvis while BWS is continually reduced. Development of trunk and pelvis stability at lower BWS is critical to translating results to the overground environment. Stand adaptability focuses on independence at the trunk and proper pelvis positioning while reducing BWS to increase weight-bearing. Challenges of reaching and squatting can be introduced (Fig. 8-5a and 8-5b).

Overground Assessment

Daily overground assessment in Phase 2 focuses primarily on trunk independence and pelvic positioning during sitting, position changes from supine to sitting (Fig. 8-6a, 8-6b, 8-6c), trunk extension, and changes from sitting to standing The therapist assesses the

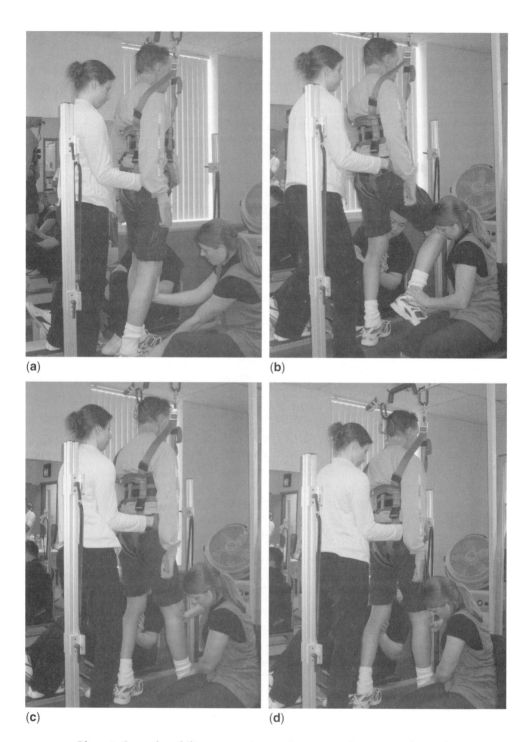

(a)

(b)

(c)

(d)

FIG 8-3 Phase 2: Step adaptability progression. **a.** Starting stride position. **b.** Stride weight shift: initial swing. **c.** Stride weight shift: heel contact. **d.** Stride weight shift: weight acceptance. Independence at trunk is achieved and independence at pelvis and then leg control are the next steps in progression.

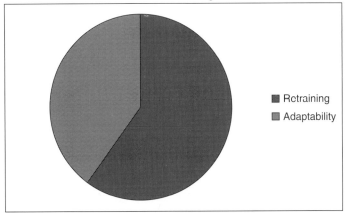

Focus of treadmill training session

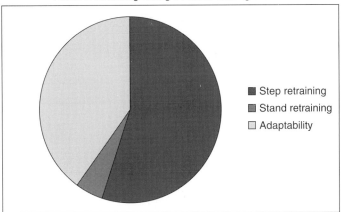

Focus of retraining during treadmill training session

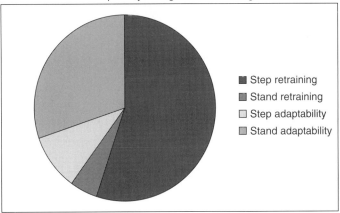

Focus of adaptability during treadmill training session

FIG 8-4 Phase 2: Approximate proportions of time spent in a training session on retraining (step and stand) and adaptability (step and stand).

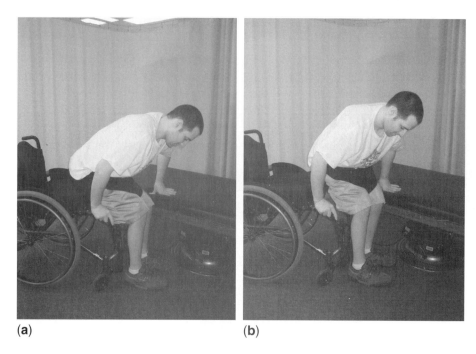

(a)   **(b)**

FIG 8-5 Phase 2: Stand adaptability progression. **a.** Stand to squat and back to stand.

client's ability to sit, stand, and balance independently for increased time durations and to shift weight laterally and in stride. The therapist assesses the client's ability, identifies the limiting factor to move forward to the next level of recovery (subphase), and makes decisions about goals for the next step training session as well as recommendations for community integration.

Community Integration

In Phase 2, the primary goals are to promote independent trunk stability and pelvis position during position changes and independent transfers with weight-bearing. The goals focus on independent standing and balancing for increased time durations and weight shifting laterally and in the stride position. Standing at home and in the community with assistance of caregivers or assistive devices is encouraged. Trainers should continue to educate the client on how to translate the Locomotor Training principles into the home/community environment, including ways to use assistive devices in a manner consistent with these principles. This could involve any activities that can load the legs, such as initiating weight-bearing (Fig. 8-7a and 8-7b) and rising to upright with a walker (Fig. 8-8a, 8-8b, 8-8c), using as much weight-bearing as possible through the legs with hip and knee extension during transfers, and standing as much as possible during daily tasks such as brushing teeth, doing dishes, and so forth. Strengthening exercises such as trunk extensions, sit-ups, reverse sit-ups, and partial-range squats should be done at home. Balance in sitting can be challenged by raising arms. The client should begin ambulation in the home and community during Phase 2c.

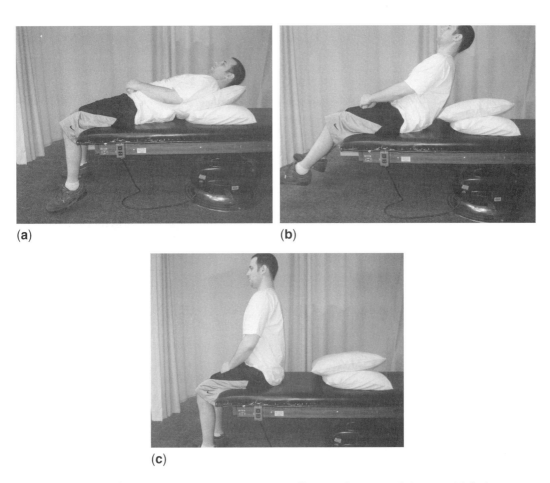

FIG 8-6 a–c. Phase 2: Sit-up progression. Using pillows to elevate trunk into partial flexion and allow practice of sit-up.

Phase 3 Progression

Clients in Phase 3 benefit by receiving Locomotor Training a minimum of three to five times per week. Their standing ability has usually been achieved, and the focus is on retraining of stepping and increasing the ability to walk overground with proper kinematics of the trunk, pelvis, and legs while decreasing dependence on assistive devices. The focus of Locomotor Training for these individuals is to become independent when transitioning from sit to stand and to increase weight-bearing and improve balance during standing. Also targeted is developing independent stepping while decreasing dependence on assistive devices, increasing weight-bearing, and improving balance. By Phase 3C, the client should be a full-time ambulator in the home and community and should be independent of assistive devices and braces. These primary goals are implemented in each component of Locomotor Training, including step training (retraining and adaptability), overground assessment (adaptability), and community integration (adaptability).

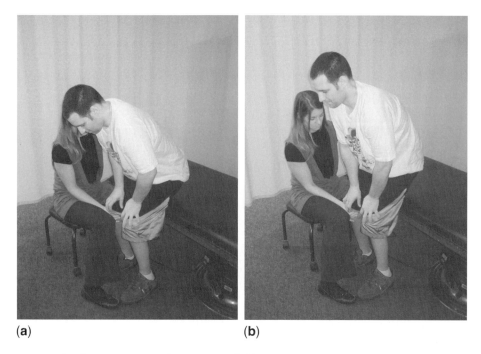

(a)   **(b)**

FIG 8-7 a, b. Phase 2: Sit to stand progression, half-stand as means to practice sit to stand using minimal weight-bearing and balance with the upper extremities.

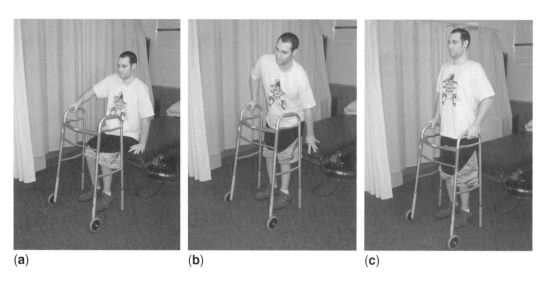

(a)   **(b)**   **(c)**

FIG 8-8 a–c. Phase 2: Community integration, sit to and from stand with a walker introduced as it may be used in the home and community.

Step Training

The primary progression of clients at Phase 3 involves maintaining good stepping endurance and speed at full weight-bearing, while progressing independence of the trunk, pelvis, and legs. During this phase, clients should be trained to repetitively reinforce the presentation of sensory cues during walking. Two or three skilled trainers (including the BWST operator) are generally required to implement the treatment intervention properly, since clients should be independent at the trunk/pelvis and may have some independence at one lower limb for a portion of the session. Trainers should continue to educate the client on how to translate the Locomotor Training principles into the home and community environment.

As the goals shift from Phase 2 to Phase 3, the focus is on increasing independence in walking and community ambulation. The total step training time is divided equally between (1) step retraining and (2) step and stand adaptability. As the client can now stand independently, retraining concentrates on step retraining. Adaptability is approximately divided between stand adaptability (about 50%) and step adaptability (about 50%, Fig. 8-9), depending on the current goals.

Step retraining emphasizes higher speeds while achieving proper kinematics with minimal manual facilitation at the pelvis, knees, and ankles at the lowest BWS levels. Stand retraining is not needed during Phase 3 of recovery because independent standing has most likely been achieved with independence at the trunk and pelvis. Step adaptability focuses on proper pelvis positioning and independence of the legs at lower BWS levels while increasing the speed of the treadmill. Adaptability should aim to maintain the progress gained in retraining while continuing to make progress with independence at the legs. To further challenge the neuromuscular system in a client who can maintain independent full weight-bearing stepping, trainers can begin to incorporate abrupt changes in speeds, inclines, and obstacle avoidance (Fig. 8-10) into the adaptability training. Stand adaptability focuses on independence at the legs while maintaining proper posture of the trunk and proper pelvis positioning at the lowest BWS levels and during challenges such as weight shifting, step-ups (Fig. 8-11), squats, single-limb standing (Fig. 8-12), and reaching tasks.

Overground Assessment

Daily overground assessment in Phase 3 focuses primarily on independent walking and pelvic positioning during transitions from supine to sitting and from sitting to standing. The therapist also assesses the client's ability to extend the trunk, independently stand with balance for increased time durations, as well as shift weight laterally and in stride (Fig. 8-13). As during step training, the client should have increased trunk/pelvis control and exhibit an alternating stepping pattern. Eventually, the client should experience walking on a variety of indoor and outdoor terrains as practice for the environments he or she will encounter in community settings. Trainers should always emphasize endurance and optimal use of the neuromuscular system.

Community Integration

In Phase 3, the primary goals are independent walking in the home and community. More than one assistive device may be used to meet varying goals, specifically endurance,

Focus of treadmill training session

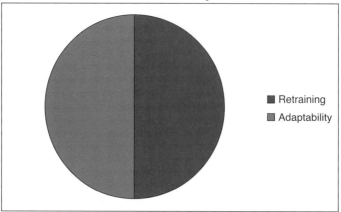

Focus of retraining during treadmill training session

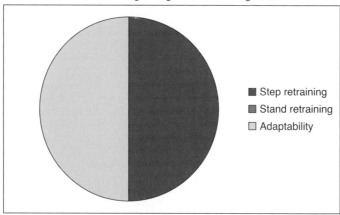

Focus of adaptability during treadmill training session

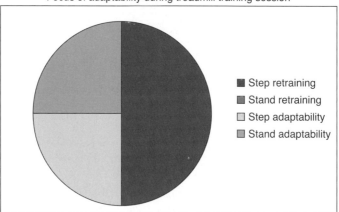

FIG 8-9 Phase 3: Approximate proportions of time spent in a training session on retraining (step and stand) and adaptability (step and stand).

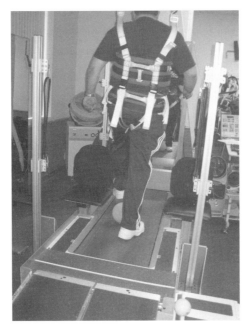

FIG 8-10 Phase 3 progression: Step adaptability. The client is avoiding the rolling obstacle on the left side of the treadmill with increased left step height and balance on the right leg.

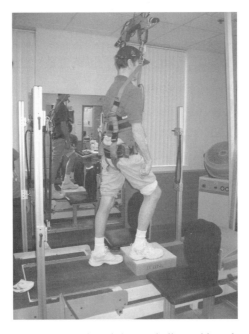

FIG 8-11 Phase 3 progression: Stand adaptability is challenged by asking client to repeatedly step up and forward onto blocks of varying heights.

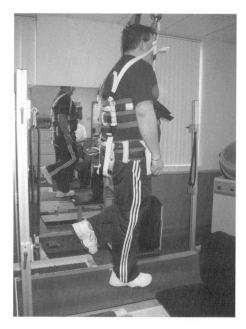

FIG 8-12 Phase 3 progression: Stand adaptability. Single-limb stance is used to challenge adaptability and balance while standing on the treadmill with body weight support.

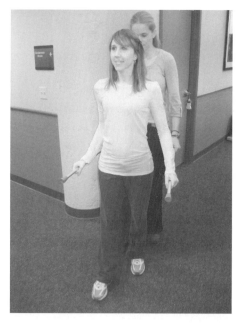

FIG 8-13 Phase 3: Overground assessment. The therapist assesses the client's ability to shift weight in stride with good trunk posture and pelvis and limb kinematics.

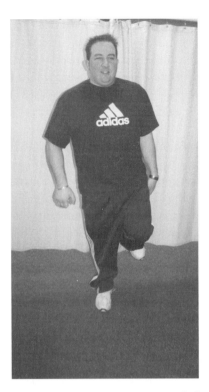

FIG 8-14 Phase 3: Community integration progression. Single-limb standing to challenge balance.

independence, appropriate kinematics (e.g., upright posture, hip extension), and activation of trunk and lower extremity muscles. The client should specifically practice walking backward for several steps. Trainers should continue to educate the client on how to translate the Locomotor Training principles to the home/community environment, including ways to use the assistive devices in a manner consistent with these principles. Strengthening exercises can include trunk extensions, sit-ups, reverse sit-ups, leg lunges similar to initiating stepping, and squats. Balance is challenged during standing by reaching, lifting, single-limb standing (Fig. 8-14), and moving the body outside the base of support. Balance is challenged during walking by walking starting and stopping, changing directions, turning around, and managing obstacles. The client should practice stair climbing, navigating curbs, and walking up and down inclines. The client should have eliminated assistive devices while walking in the home and community during Phase 3c.

Phase 4 Progression

Clients in the final stage of recovery should focus on increasing endurance with no use of devices, decrease any gait deviations at higher speeds, and be able to adapt to the environmental and behavioral demands of walking in the home and community (i.e., obstacle negotiation, speed changes, stairs, dual tasks). In addition, recreational activities requiring walking and running may be used to set progression goals. By the end of Phase 4, the client should be a full-time ambulator in the community with the ability to adjust to speed changes, negotiate uneven terrain, walk long distances, and maintain balance on uneven terrain or unpredictable circumstances or during dual tasks (e.g., walking and carrying an item). In addition, the client will be able to run safely for recreational purposes.

Step Training

The primary progression of Phase 4 step training is to further challenge the neuromuscular system in a client who can already maintain independent full weight-bearing stepping at endurance levels for community mobility. During this phase, clients should be trained with intermittent and varied conditions, both predictable and unpredictable: various speeds, inclines and obstacle avoidance, starts/stops, and dual tasking (verbal and manual). One or three skilled trainers (including the BWST operator) are generally required to implement the treatment intervention properly, since clients should be independent at the trunk/pelvis and may have some independence at the legs for a portion of the session. During this phase, clients should be trained three times per week.

In Phase 4, the client's walking function may appear very similar on the treadmill and overground, with no BWS and no manual assistance, and he or she should be able to walk independently with a good kinematic pattern at pre-injury speeds. The step training environment emphasizes pursuing goals relative to adaptability. The focus is on challenging the client's ability to adapt his or her locomotor pattern to the demands of the predictable and unpredictable community environments and to meet both recreational and personal goals.

Step retraining goals emphasize good stepping endurance at high speeds and at full weight-bearing, while progressing independence during running. Recreational pursuits such as running can be safely practiced during step training. Stand retraining and stand adaptability are not required. Step adaptability should further challenge the neuromuscular system in a client who can maintain independent full weight-bearing stepping and who can begin to incorporate various speeds, inclines, and obstacle avoidance into the adaptability training. In this environment the client can experience the limits of his or her abilities for dynamic balance and adaptation of walking without the fear of falling. With the safety in place, recovery from stumbles can be practiced without falls.

Overground Assessment

Daily overground assessment in Phase 4 focuses on achieving supine to sit-up, reverse sit-ups, trunk extensions, and sit to stand similar to the client's pre-injury abilities. Independent standing and walking is dynamic and the client is able to balance without an assistive device even when challenged.

Community Integration

In Phase 4, the primary goals include independent walking on a variety of indoor and outdoor terrains. The client should seek task demands that challenge his or her current skill set for community ambulation (e.g., curbs, stairs [with/without a rail], inclines, uneven terrain, carrying objects, turning around, opening doors) (Fig. 8-15). The client should practice walking in complex situations at home, at work, or during leisure activities (e.g., pushing a stroller, walking hand in hand with a child or partner, walking a dog,

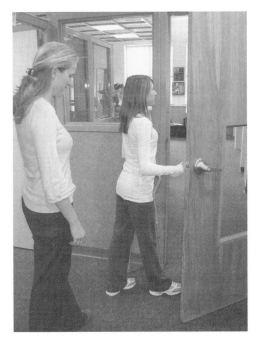

FIG 8-15 Phase 3: Community integration progression. Client challenges walking and balance skills by opening door.

carrying groceries [Fig. 8-16], walking with a backpack, pushing a heavy cart [Fig. 8-17], stepping onto an escalator, or climbing a ladder [Fig. 8-18]). The client is encouraged to return to pre-injury leisure and recreational activities and to explore new activities. To do so may require community-based instruction specific to the goal (e.g., kayaking, karate, fishing) but may also inform the therapist of goal-specific needs for improved neuromuscular control.

Overall Summary

The ultimate success of the Locomotor Training intervention is highly dependent on the quality of the step retraining, the intensity of the treatment, continuous challenges provided to the client to progress, and the decisions made by the clinician regarding the progression. The clinician should identify the three lowest-scored items of the Phase of Recovery and focus the immediate goals on reaching the next level. The step and stand retraining emphasizes providing the appropriate sensory cues for the motor task repetitively to drive plasticity of the nervous system. As the neuromuscular system's potential increases, then the client and clinician can adapt the new capacity to achieving functional goals in daily life. The clinician now has access to additional tools to improve functional recovery due to better understanding of the circuitry of the human spinal cord. Locomotor Training principles can be applied to neurologic disorders or diseases that do not directly damage the lumbosacral spinal cord. Thus, the general approach to provide

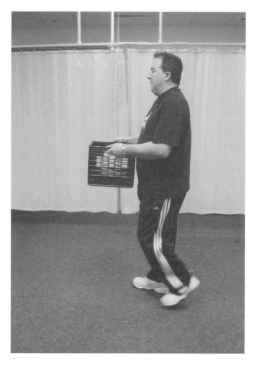

FIG 8-16 Phase 4: Community integration. The client's balance while walking is challenged by carrying a crate.

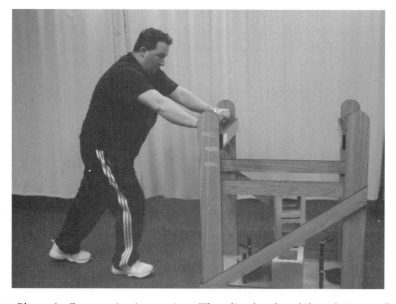

FIG 8-17 Phase 4: Community integration. The client's adaptability during walking is challenged by the additional task of pushing a weighted sled.

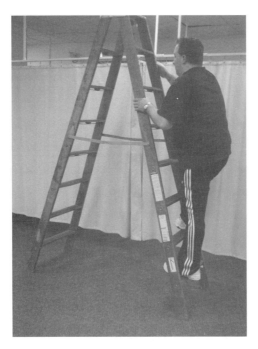

FIG 8-18 Phase 4: Community integration progression. Tasks that require walking and that were performed pre-injury in the home and community are identified. In this instance, the client practiced climbing a ladder.

the intervention is the same regardless of the pathology or whether the injury occurs in the brain or the cervical or thoracic spinal cord.

Scientific and clinical evidence is continuously emerging, and the information presented here is based on current knowledge. Clinicians are highly encouraged to continue to review the literature and evidence for activity-based therapies and continue to enrich their clinical practice to improve the functional outcomes after neurologic injury. A new era has emerged for those who suffer from paralysis in which higher achievements of function, overall health improvements, and a better quality of life can be realized.

Index

Note: Page numbers followed by "*f*" and "*t*" denote figures and tables, respectively.